Oska Guttmann

Aesthetic Physical Culture

A self-instructor for all cultured circles, and especially for oratorical and dramatic

artists

Oska Guttmann

Aesthetic Physical Culture
A self-instructor for all cultured circles, and especially for oratorical and dramatic artists

ISBN/EAN: 9783337304133

Printed in Europe, USA, Canada, Australia, Japan

Cover: Foto ©Thomas Meinert / pixelio.de

More available books at **www.hansebooks.com**

ÆSTHETIC PHYSICAL CULTURE.

A SELF-INSTRUCTOR

FOR

ALL CULTURED CIRCLES, AND ESPECIALLY FOR ORATORICAL AND DRAMATIC ARTISTS.

BY

OSKAR GUTTMANN,

PROFESSOR OF ÆSTHETIC PHYSICAL CULTURE, VOICE-PRODUCTION, ORATORY, DRAMATIC
READING AND ACTING; AUTHOR OF "GYMNASTICS OF THE VOICE"
"TALENT AND SCHOOL," ETC., ETC

ORIGINAL ILLUSTRATIONS

ALBANY, N. Y.:
EDGAR S. WERNER,
The Voice Press,
1884.

PREFACE TO THE FIRST GERMAN EDITION.

> We all, as respects our knowledge and abilities, stand upon the experience of earlier races; and popular progress could not be imaginable if we treated the arts and sciences as mere empirics.
> A. CZERWINSKI in "The History of Dancing."

Among the ancient Greeks, all gymnastic exercises, and especially dancing, formed a leading element of the education of youth. Solon, the lawgiver, ordained the study of gymnastics; and Pythagoras, the founder of a rational system, won the applause of the populace as a gymnast. High and low, old and young, cultivated this art. According to Plato, the man who found no pleasure in dancing and gymnastics, was a rude, unpolished clown. The great value the Greeks placed upon these two arts, is evident from their assiduous cultivation by the greatest men: poets, generals, and sages. Sophocles and Epaminondas were renowned dancers, and Socrates did not think it undignified to zealously practice dancing in his old age, because he thought that it contributed to outward and inward symmetry. There were also great poets in those days, who were masters of the art of dancing. Arion, Tyrtæus, as well as Æschylus, won great repute by their gestures and dancing. The utmost modesty in glance and demeanor was in that day considered an absolute necessity, and a rapid gait was not "good form." Demosthenes placed bold speech and a rapid gait in the same category. The ancient Hellenes went so far as to judge of a man's character by his gait and movements.

With the fall of Greece, a rough athletism took the place of the noble principles of Pythagoras. Toward the end of the Grecian rule this culminated, and then passed over to the Romans, who witnessed with rapturous applause combats between men and wild beasts, or mortal conflicts between man and man, where, while the dead gladiator was ignominiously dragged from the arena, the victor received the branch of palm, and was often rewarded with money.

The following example will show what a strict difference the Grecians, in the palmy days of their empire, made between rational gymnastics and the rough antics of athletes and gymnasts:

"To Clisthenes came Hippoclides, the son of Pisandros, a rich Greek, to sue for the hand of his daughter. The father consented. When, at a family feast at which gymnastic sports were usually carried on, Hippoclides, through leaping and other antics, hoped still more to win the favor of the father of his Agarista, and at last, after all possible masterpieces, placed himself upon his head and began to gesticulate with his legs as if they were arms, Clisthenes, long since enraged at these absurd performances, cried out: 'O, son of Pisandros, thou hast danced away thy marriage!'

In Rome, where, as we have seen, gymnastics degenerated into horrible cruelties, the dance rose at length to great popularity in spite of the opposition of almost all the renowned authors and statesmen. After the introduction of the Greek play, which was a musical declamatory representation, and in which, for the Roman public, dancing and music were the main things, the dancer Dionysia received an income of 42,000 marks,* and the renowned actor Roscius, a contemporary of Cicero, an income of 129,000 marks.

After the fall of Rome there is a chasm of many centuries in the history of gymnastics.

In the middle ages, it was the tournament that demanded skill and decorum as well as strength. After the fall of the tournament, scarce anything was done for physical culture, and only with the Reformation, with Luther himself, does the time begin anew in which the necessity of making mind and body symmetrical, was recognized. Montaigne, the French essayist (born 1533), says: "I would have an outward decorum and pleasing manners cultivated at the same time with the mind. It

---

* The former over $10,000 in our money, the latter nearly $33,000. — *Translator*.

Preface to the First German Edition.

is not a soul, not a body, we educate; it is a man. Out of this one we must not make two." And Plato says: "We must not break in one without the other; but must urge and guide both alike, like a span of horses harnessed to a shaft."

In the seventeenth and eighteenth centuries, there were special dancing-masters who taught deportment and fine manners to grown persons and to children, dancing being considered the basis of all good manners, since more grace entailed greater decorum. And where were more elegance, more grace in gait and bearing necessary than in a court minuet, or gavotte? An age when gallants wore embroidered garments, and carried swords, enforced a strict attention to the outward proprieties, and to fine manners.

That race is no more. The time has gone by when a Marcel, the most renowned of European ballet-masters (his lessons cost very dear, he being paid 300 francs for the bow to be made at a court presentation, or for a minuet to be danced at some state ball), — could say to one duchess: "Madame, your courtsey is like that of a maid-servant;" and to another: "You have a gait like a fish-wife. Lay aside these wretched manners and begin your bows anew, never forgetting what you are, and that a consciousness of your rank should control your slightest actions."* Lord Chesterfield urgently exhorted his son to take lessons of Marcel in deportment, so that he might enter a *salon* without any awkward movements of the arms or body; and, upon his first introduction to society, produce a favorable impression which would be likely to endure.

The age is now gone by when Louis XIV. took dancing-lessons twenty years in order to perfect himself in the minuet and gavotte, where the finest grace must have expression. Those days are past, and those dancing-masters have left no successors. Were there any such, they might starve for lack of pupils; for, as the public announcements tell us daily, all society-dances may be learned in eight hours, and few are willing to give more time

---

* Czerwinski's "History of Dancing."

than this. In no society of the present day, at no court, it might almost be said, is a strict etiquette observed.

Modern *turnerei*, with its bold antics, its gigantic leaps, and contortions of the body, is far removed from the rational gymnastics of Pythagoras, and not calculated to produce decorum or grace.

Where shall the youth or the maiden learn anything of deportment? A book should be written from which our young people, anxious for fine manners, may draw counsel. So-called books of etiquette to-day, where everything is reduced to a science, aid, at most, only in attaining a superficial polish. Even a work on decorum must have a strict scientific basis, if it would answer its purpose, if it would be abreast of the times, and take due account of the laws of æsthetics.

Much has been written upon decorum and fine manners. Even our most renowned authorities, such as Goethe, have expressed their ideas upon this subject; but we nowhere find a system, a perfect method. We possess works upon gymnastics, dancing, fencing, the plastic and histrionic arts, etc., but none in which, out of all these, a system is deduced, from which true culture may be derived.

German literature has, indeed, for several years, been enriched by a work which must be placed in quite another category, and for which we have to thank the talent and tireless industry of Herr Hugo Rothstein, Director of the Prussian Royal Central School of Gymnastics. This is an excellent adaptation of the celebrated work of Ling, a Swedish teacher of gymnastics and father of the modern rational science of that name. Its title is *Gymnastics*. But, excellent as the work is, its benefits must be derived indirectly through the teacher; it would be useless for the pupil to seek to master a work comprising five volumes, and over 1600 pages.

If we turn to the literature of the mimic art, we find ourselves in the same dilemma. This literature is very comprehensive, and embraces much that is valuable, from Quintilian down to

Preface to the First German Edition. vii

writers of our own day; but all these works, in spite of their many excellences, lack one fundamental thing: Instruction in training the limbs to a capability for the mimic art, without which all advice is useless.

The main requirement in the mimic art is to have the body as a whole, and its members severally, so in one's power that the moods of the soul may be easily and gracefully rendered. No treatise upon acting can teach that art by merely laying down rules how to give intellectual expression to our passions; quite apart from the fact that the ways in which our passions may be expressed are so manifold, and so distinct, that it would be almost impossible to establish fixed rules. There can be no real acting until the limbs and the body, as a whole, are made so elastic by training that the physical movements express æsthetically the disposition of the soul.

Hegel says: "My body is the medium through which I communicate with the outward world. If I would realize my intention, I must make myself capable of rendering this subjectivity into outward objectivity. My body is not naturally fitted for this; it conforms only to the physical life. The organic and physical impulses are not yet the results of the promptings of my spirit. My body must first be trained for such service." And Dr. Jacobs expresses the idea of Greek gymnastics by saying that their one great aim was to secure the mastery of mind over body, and represent the internal harmony in the inward and outward appearance.

After these words no especial proof is needed to show that the method of studying certain fixed movements for this or that situation, this or that sensation, — a method adopted by many teachers, — is false and execrable. It should, on the contrary, be our task to make the body so elastic, so strictly subject to the will by correct, regular, and varied practice, that, if we would reproduce a sensation, we may make as through an electric shock, not a certain or fixed, but yet an appropriate movement of the limbs; for varied and still befitting gestures may be made for every expression. When we are sure that the movements of the limbs are round and pleasing, we can safely trust ourselves to our sensations, certain that these will be truly and beautifully expressed.

Then the study of the mimic art must not begin until this point of culture has been reached by careful study.

Who would recommend a teacher of harmony to a talented young musician before he can play well upon some instrument? Who would mention tactics and strategy to a soldier before he has learned the first evolutions, or advise the art-student to employ a teacher in color before he has learned to draw? The fundamental elements of every science and art must be studied first, and the basis of acting is gymnastics — not in the strictly pedagogic (physical) sense, but gymnastics with strict regard to æsthetics and to the plastic movements of the body.

The reason for the lack of such a basis in the literature of this subject, is the supposition of the authors that first principles have been acquired in youth, and before the student began to practice art. But this is a false supposition.

Aside from the fact that but few are able to give the body gymnastic culture in youth, and that most pursue callings apart from such culture before they go upon the stage, — aside from all this, no mere pedagogic physical system will suffice for acting. A system of gymnastics written for the health, is far removed from inculcating charm and grace. While it treats of the limbs with especial reference to strength and movement, æsthetic gymnastics demand the cultivation of the limbs to a harmonious whole, exact regard for æsthetic personation, and that, too, in one perfected system.

Æsthetic gymnastics, therefore, form the a, b, c of acting, and without them a knowledge of the latter art is no more possible than to learn a language without knowing the alphabet. But, as without æsthetic gymnastics, acting is impossible, so there can be no æsthetic instruction without a previous course of physical gymnastics. And, again, a knowledge of the outlines of anatomy, at least, is indispensable to the correct and healthful practice of gymnastics. This knowledge of the art of acting must, then, be preceded by some acquaintance with human anatomy and physiology, with physical and æsthetic gymnastics.

Then only is the student capable of grasping the principles of acting. We say the principles, for more than these we regard as superfluous and impracticable, because acting is the outcome of the active soul, and this in a body æsthetically cultured, finds a right way of itself.

"Who can undertake," says Professor Harless in his excellent work entitled *Plastic Anatomy*, — "who can undertake to analyze and reproduce in word and picture for the use of the artist, the endless number of movements and poses which we assume involuntarily, or to which an inner impulse urges us with mysterious power? Only one way remains, but that suffices for the true artist. He whose heart and understanding, guided by a thorough culture of the intellect, are in a condition to trace out the profound emotions of the soul-life, to search sharply into the motives of human actions, and to follow sympathetically the experiences of various cultivated men, — for such an one it suffices to know those various and easily understood views and proclivities which, arising within the mind, now in this, now in that connection, return ever and ever again to allow themselves to be expressed in pantomime."

Hence it is evident that a work which assumes the task of laying down rules for mental activity to the minutest degree, will prove useless, and that even an exposition of the mere principles of the mimic art will bear little fruit if the above-named conditions of previous study are wanting.

Long years' practice of the dramatic art, as well as of physical and æsthetic gymnastics, many years of imparting instruction in both, combined with profound study of all works pertaining to the subject, justify me, I think, in attempting to write such a work for the stage and for the public. I call my work an attempt, but whether it will be more than this, whether it will be as kindly received as my *Gymnastics of the Voice*, the future must decide.

In any event, the student will recognize in my work a most profound devotion to a calling designed to cultivate and ennoble men. As in my *Gymnastics of the Voice*, I have only given the methods of forming a correct tone, and of correctly articulating the alphabet, (the basis of the arts of singing and rhetoric), — so in this book I have only given a basis to the works already written upon the mimic art, in order to make them available for the actor, and set forth the principles of the æsthetic culture of the human body. If I succeed in this effort, I shall feel myself rewarded.

An acquaintance with dancing and fencing being indispensable to physical culture, I have taken up the principles of both arts, and besides added a treatise upon the laws of dress, ending with rules for social life in its everyday walks and in the *salon*, embodied in a special chapter.

Those whose youth was so highly favored that they learned systematically all those things which give the body its highest elasticity and strength (such as wrestling, swimming, fencing, dancing, riding, gymnastic exercises, etc.), will find my book of less interest, although they, too, will discover many things, either entirely new, or at least new in their thoroughness. Those who belong to public life, but had no opportunities for youthful culture, will find the work indispensable, while it will prove useful to people in private life, since it is impossible to obtain perfect mastery of the limbs without systematic practice, and to avoid faults in movement without a study and comprehension of the principles of gymnastics.

Tyros are too apt to think that with a few years practice on the stage, ease of movement, a correct action of the limbs and all minor accessories will come of themselves As well might the raw recruit who goes weighted with pack and knapsack and without preparatory discipline into battle, think to discharge his duty as well as he who has thoroughly learned the military tactics.

The wood-engravings which accompany this work have all been drawn from nature with the greatest care by the painter Fratrel, in accordance with instructions and illustrations from the author.

PREFACE TO THE FIRST GERMAN EDITION.

Should any one find that I have omitted to speak on subjects, especially on those pertaining to the domain of Æsthetic Gymnastics, I should be pleased to have them pointed out by letter. I will gladly answer such communications, as far as time allows, and will treat of them in a future edition, should one be granted me.

OSKAR GUTTMANN,
Manager of the Stadt Theatre.
Hamburg (Germany), 1865.

PREFACE TO THE SECOND GERMAN EDITION.

"I call my work an attempt, but whether it will be more than this, whether it will be as kindly received as my *Gymnastics of the Voice*, the future must decide."

With these words I sent the first edition of this book out into the world. It was, however, received with extraordinary favor. Critics praised it and leading journals gave extended notices and testimonials. This was proof sufficient that *Æsthetic Physical Culture* supplied a want and was a necessary work.

Notwithstanding this unanimous recognition of my efforts, I still did not feel satisfied. I knew only too well that I had not attained unto what I had striven for; yes, indeed, that the full realization of my purpose was almost an impossibility, as the subject is inexhaustible. But what could I do? At that time I no more thought of a second edition of this book than I did at the first edition of my *Gymnastics of the Voice*, and so I had to submit.

But it turned out otherwise. Notwithstanding its imperfections, *Æsthetic Physical Culture* proved such a useful book that a second edition became necessary. I undertook the revision with all the heart, with all the love, with all the holy earnestness with which I had devoted my whole life to dramatic art.

The whole text has been revised and rewritten. Much of the first edition has been enlarged upon and given again in plainer terms. Large additions of new material have been made, the result of constant study of and instruction in the principles and requirements of the drama.

Works upon the mimic art abound, and it would be difficult to produce anything new or better in this department of literature. But, so far as I know, nothing similar to *Æsthetic Physical Culture* exists,—a book that in a rational, scientific, practical manner gives the means by which the body and its movements can be æsthetically trained, and the scholar prepared to enter upon the study of the mimic art.

PREFACE TO THE SECOND GERMAN EDITION. xiii

Now and then I have heard it remarked, "The study of the book and the following of its teachings is too difficult!" Much as I may regret it, I can not make it easier. The only consolation I find is in the words of Friederich Spielhagen, who, in reviewing my book in the *Sonntagsblatt*, said : "Those, who believe they can accomplish everything through talent alone, without study, may exclaim, after examining the book, 'The obstacles are insurmountable!' and make no further attempt. Such persons would do well to abandon the dramatic profession, for energy and perseverance are qualities indispensable to the artist."

I fully agree with the criticism of the Hamburg *Reform*, viz., that "Part Third is the kernel of the whole book, and should be studied by all dramatic and oratorical students, not, however, before the first two parts have been thoroughly mastered. Indeed, it is a carefully graded text-book no part of which can be omitted, if good results are desired."

So, I now send this new, improved and enlarged edition over the ocean, to my old home, among the ranks of those who are sincerely striving to place dramatic instruction upon a systematic, scientific basis. May *Æsthetic Physical Culture* contribute its mite to that end !

I take leave of my readers in quoting the words used by Dr. Feodor Wehl in concluding his review of the first edition of this book :

"May the entire dramatic profession and all other persons of artistic vocations or natures cordially welcome this book. By so doing they will themselves be benefited and also promote dramatic and oratorical art."

THE AUTHOR.

New York, 1879.

PREFACE TO THE AMERICAN EDITION.

In presenting *Æsthetic Physical Culture* in the language of my adopted country, nothing need be added to the preceding prefaces, which tell the story of the book and explain its scope. I can only wish that it may be as cordially received by the American public as it was in my native land.

OSKAR GUTTMANN,

436 East 57th st., New York.

1884.

CONTENTS.

PART FIRST.

ANATOMICAL AND PHYSIOLOGICAL PRINCIPLES.

THE HUMAN SKELETON.
    The Bones of the Head.................................... 4
    The Torso... 4
    The Upper Limbs.. 6
    The Lower Limbs.. 6

THE MUSCLES.
    The Muscles of the Head................................. 12
    The Muscles of the Face................................. 12
    The Muscles of the Torso................................ 13
    The Muscles of the Upper Limbs.......................... 13
    The Muscles of the Lower Limbs.......................... 14

THE MECHANISM OF THE LIMBS.
    The Centre of Gravity................................... 15
    The Mechanism of the Walking Apparatus.................. 18
    Walking Forward... 22
    Walking Backward.. 23

PART SECOND.

PHYSICAL GYMNASTICS.

INTRODUCTION.
    Directions for Practice................................. 27

THE SINGLE MEMBERS—SIMPLE EXERCISES.
    Base Position... 30
    Turning the Head to the Right and Left.................. 31

CONTENTS.

Bowing of the Head Forward, Backward, or to the Right and Left ... 31
The Head Circle ... 31
Shoulder Movements ... 32
The Shoulder Circle ... 33
Rising and Falling of the Hips ... 34
Turning or Twisting of the Trunk ... 34
Inclination of the Torso Forward, Backward, Right and Left ... 34
The Torso Circle ... 35
Elevating the Torso ... 35
Arm Exercises ... 36

ARM EXERCISES WITH OUTSTRETCHED ARMS.
Lifting and Moving the Arm ... 37
The Arm Circle ... 37
Turning and Revolving the Arms ... 37
Balancing and Oblique Movements ... 38

ARM EXERCISES WITH THE AID OF THE ELBOW-JOINTS.
Attraction and Repulsion ... 39
Movement of the Arms behind the Back ... 40

HAND AND WRIST PRACTICE.
Finger-Stretching and Spreading ... 41

LEG AND FOOT PRACTICE.
Exercise with Stretched Leg—Leg Swinging ... 42
The Leg Circle, Forward and Backward ... 43
The Flexion and Extension of the Knee Backward ... 43
The Flexion and Extension of the Knee Forward ... 43
Strengthening of the Muscles of the Legs ... 44
Foot Extension ... 45
Foot Extension, Flexion and Circling ... 46

THE LIMBS AS A WHOLE—COMPLEX EXERCISES.
Exercises for the Upper Part of the Body ... 47
Exercises for the Legs and Feet—The "Leg Circle" ... 50
Exercises for the Upper Body, Legs and Feet ... 51

PART THIRD.

ÆSTHETIC GYMNASTICS.

INTRODUCTION.
THE PLASTIC ART.
The Human Body and its Limbs ... 58

CONTENTS.

    The Limbs Singly, in a State of Rest........................ 58
    Movement of the Arms and Hands........................ 62

MOVEMENTS.
    Walking in General.. 73
    The Walking of Ladies with Trains........................ 73
    The Lifting of a Lady's Dress in Walking................. 75
    Turning to the Right or Left in Walking................. 75
    Turning to the Right or Left While Standing.............. 75
    Walking Sideward... 75
    Stepping Sideward With Bowing........................... 76
    Turning Round in Walking................................. 76
    Turning Round While Standing............................. 77
    Turning in the Case of Women............................. 77
    Carriage of the Arms in Walking.......................... 78
    The Opening of a Door.................................... 78
    The Entrance of a Servant................................ 79
    The Setting of a Chair for One's Self or for Others...... 79
    Seating One's Self upon a Chair already Placed........... 80
    Kneeling... 82
    Lifting Something from the Floor......................... 84
    Falling upon the Stage................................... 84
    The Holding of the Hat................................... 85
    The Carrying of the Fan.................................. 86
    The Carrying of a Cane................................... 87
    The Use of the Handkerchief.............................. 88
    The Hand-Kiss.. 89
    Fundamental Rules for Position if Several Persons are on the Stage... 90
    Position of Subordinates................................. 92

THE MIMIC ART.
PLAY OF FEATURES.
    General Remarks.. 93
    The Eyes... 94
    The Mouth.. 95
    Main Elements of Facial Expression....................... 97

GENERAL PHYSIOGNOMICAL REMARKS.
    The Cheeks... 103
    The Lips... 103
    The Chin... 103

GESTURE.
THE SINGLE LIMBS IN RELATION TO GESTURE.
The Head.. 104
The Arms and Hands in General......................... 106
Main Principles of the Position of the Hand in Acting........ 109
The Torso... 111
The Legs and Feet.. 112
Walking in Acting... 114
Characteristic Tokens of Several Kinds of Gait.............. 115

THE LIMBS IN HARMONIOUS ACTION.
The Divisions of Gesture.................................. 117
The Fundamental Rules for Correct Action of the Limbs in Gesture... 119
The Use of the Left and Right Hand...................... 122
Greeting, Prayer, Oath.................................... 123
Salutations of the Hebrews................................ 124
The Moslem Salutation.................................... 125
Chinese Salutations....................................... 127
Salutations of the Hindoos, Greeks and Romans............ 128
Salutation, Oath and Prayer of Modern Times According to the European Fashion among Civilized People............. 129

VARIOUS FAULTY GESTURES AND THEIR CORRECTION.
Drinking.. 130
The Holding of a Cup of Coffee or Tea.................... 131
Pantomimic Reading and Letter Writing..................... 131
Turning the Leaves of a Book............................. 133
Use of a Pencil... 133
Practical Exercises for Pupils............................. 133

PART FOURTH.
THE ART OF DANCING.

THE ART OF DANCING.
Carriage of the Body..................................... 139
Fundamental Positions and Movements...................... 140
The Position of the Feet.................................. 140
The Position of the Arms.................................. 142
Exercises Preliminary to the Dance........................ 144
Single Movements of the Feet through which the Dancing Steps are Rendered Possible........................... 147

CONTENTS. xix

Elementary Dancing Steps........................... 147
Composite Independent Steps......................... 150
The Minuet as a School for Compliments............... 151

COMPLIMENT—REVERENCE.

The Compliment of Ancient Times.................... 152
The Mediæval Compliment. 152
The Compliment of the 17th and 18th Centuries........ 153
The Great Reverence for Gentlemen................... 154
The Great Reverence for Ladies...................... 156
The Little Reverence for Gentlemen................... 158
The Little Reverence for Ladies...................... 159
Reverence before Several Persons Standing in a Half-Circle... 160
The Little Reverence upon Arrival and at Departure, also at
    Meeting in Walking, for Gentlemen and for Ladies.. 161–162
The Modern Compliment............................ 163

PART FIFTH.
THE ART OF FENCING.

THE ART OF FENCING.

The Foil... 169
The Measure...................................... 169
Place and Position................................. 170
First Position..................................... 170
Second Position................................... 171
Attitude of the Hand............................... 172
The Foot Movement................................ 174
The Primary Thrust................................ 176
The Secondary Thrust.............................. 177
Simple Parades.................................... 178
Counter-Parades................................... 178
The Dégagement................................... 179
The Doublé....................................... 179
The Coupé.. 179
Compliment of Arms............................... 179
General Advice.................................... 181

PART SIXTH.

MAIN PRINCIPLES OF DRESS.

MAIN PRINCIPLES OF DRESS.
    Women's Dress.. 185
    Men's Dress... 188
    Combination of Colors... 191

PART SEVENTH.

APPLICATION OF THE RULES TO COMMON LIFE, THE SALON AND THE STAGE.

APPLICATION OF THE RULES.
    What is Decorum?... 197
    Politeness and Modesty.. 198
    Deportment toward Ladies....................................... 202
    Deportment in Large Companies................................. 203
    Deportment at a Ball.. 205
    Deportment at Table.. 208
    Deportment at the Theatre or Concert........................... 210
    The Visit of Ceremony.. 211
    Audience with Princes.. 212
    The Manner of Studying this Book without a Teacher............ 213

PART FIRST.

ANATOMICAL AND PHYSIOLOGICAL PRINCIPLES.

"The thought originates in the brain, the brain acts upon the nerves, the nerves upon the muscles, the muscles upon the bones, and not until after this process is it possible for us to undertake any action."

GUTTMANN'S "Gymnastics of the Voice."

CHAPTER I.

THE HUMAN SKELETON.

The skeleton of the human body is composed of bones and cartilages, united by flexible cords, and forming a movable apparatus which can be set in action by the muscles. The peculiar articulation of the bones gives rise to cavities within the skeleton (the cavities of the head, brain, chest, abdomen and pelvis), in which the various internal organs, designed partly for nourishment and partly for mental activity, have their seat. All these parts are permeated by greater or smaller veins, and by white fibres: the former, the arteries, carry the blood from the heart through the body, and again back to the heart; and the latter, the white fibres or nerves, bind the different parts of the body into one harmonious whole. They proceed from the brain and the spinal marrow, and, excited by outward or inward impulse, cause motion, sensation, and intellectual activity. As long as man lives, a constant change is going on in the particles which compose his body, and this forces him to take the necessary food.

Physical gymnastics teach the laws through whose observance this change may go on regularly and advantageously. The office of *æsthetic gymnastics* is to make the limbs appear graceful and pleasing in accordance with *æsthetic laws*.

The greater divisions of the human body are the *head*, *trunk* and *limbs*. The *head*, the upper and most important part, is movably set upon the neck, and contains the brain in its upper half, while its lower half forms the face, with cavities for the organs of the senses. The *trunk* or *torso* is divided into four parts, — the neck, the chest, the abdomen and pelvis, and has its support in the spinal column. The front of the neck contains the organs of the voice, and the air and food tubes. The chest contains the breathing apparatus and the heart. The abdomen and pelvis contain the sustaining and reproductive organs. The limbs, which enclose no vital organ, are bordered with muscles, and may be divided into two groups: The *upper* limbs, the arms, which consist of the shoulder, the upper arm, and the lower arm and hand, are joined to the chest by ligaments, while the *lower* limbs, the legs — consisting of the upper and lower leg and the foot, — are joined by ligaments to the pelvis.

The single bones of these main groups are:

1. The Bones of the Head

Consisting of the skull and the face. The skull is composed of eight bones, firmly and elaborately united; the face of fourteen bones, only one of which, the lower jaw, is movable, while the upper bones, like those of the skull, are bound strongly together.

2. The Torso.

This has its main support in the backbone or spinal column. It consists of twenty-six single bones. The seven upper ones (Fig. I., 1–7) are the bones of the neck; the next twelve (8–20) are the breast and backbones; and the five lower ones (21–26) belong to the abdomen and loins, and unite with the os sacrum (26) and coccyx (27), which form the terminal extremity of the spinal column. On each side of the twelve breastbones, and united with them, stand twelve rib-bones (8–19), which are in turn joined by tendons to the breastbone (28). In this way is formed the chest-cavity which contains those important organs, the heart and lungs. By means of muscles fastened to these bones, the chest-cavity may be expanded or contracted, whereby the breathing process is mainly carried on. Upon each side of the sacrum (29–30) lies a bone of the pelvis, whose upper surface is called the hip-bone. The pelvis-cavity is composed of four bones, — the two innominata, the sacrum and the coccyx. The abdominal cavity lies between that of the pelvis

THE HUMAN SKELETON.

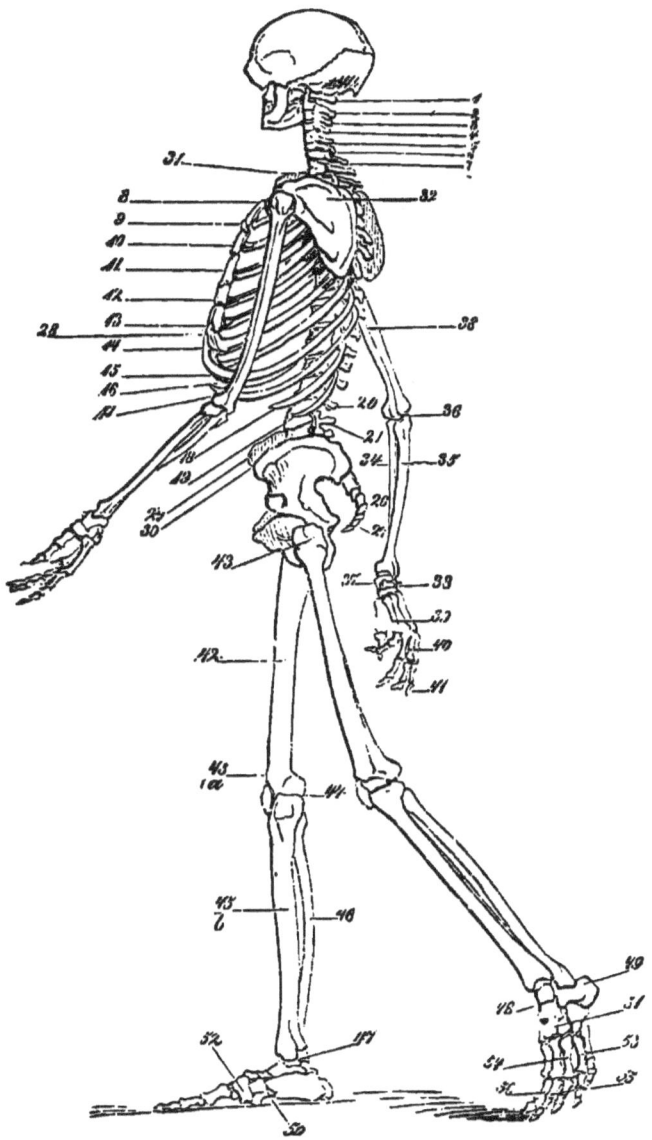

Fig. I.

and the chest, and is the seat of the greater portion of the digestive organs.

3. *The Upper Limbs, or the Arms.*

These consist of the shoulder, the shoulder-joint, the humerus or upper arm, the lower arm and the hand. The hand consists of the wrist, the palm and the fingers. The shoulder-bones consist of the two clavicles, or collar-bones (31) and the shoulder-blades (32). The first extend from the breastbone to the shoulder-joint; the latter lie along the back, connecting with the clavicles and bones of the upper arms, and forming the shoulder-joints. By means of the clavicles, which, as we have said, connect the bones of the humerus with the torso, the shoulder-joint is held at the required distance from the torso, and the arms receive the necessary freedom in their movements. The bone of the upper arm (33), which is joined to the shoulder-blade and to the two bones of the lower arm, helps in this way to form the shoulder and elbow-joint. The lower arm has two bones, the radius (34) and the ulna (35). The junction of the upper and lower arm forms the elbow-joint (36). The wrist is composed of eight bones, ranged in two rows, and bound firmly together. The five bones of the metacarpus, or middle hand, articulate with the second range of carpal bones (39). The four fingers and the thumb articulate with these five metacarpal bones, the thumb having two joints and the fingers three, the first of which is the largest (40), the lower (41) being called the nail-joint.

4. *The Lower Limbs, or the Legs*

Consist of the upper leg, the lower leg and the foot. The upper leg, like the upper arm, has but one bone, the femur (42). At its top there is a ball-shaped joint (43) which fits into the socket of the pelvis, and forms the hip-joint. At its lower end it connects with the shin-bone and the knee-pan, forming the knee-joint (44). The knee-pan (45 *a*) is a heart-shaped bone which covers the front part of the cavity of the knee-joint, and is attached to the bones of both the upper and lower leg.

The lower leg, like the lower arm, consists of two bones, the tibia (45 *b*) and the fibula (46). The first is much larger than the second. At the lower end of these bones (47) are joints connecting them with the foot, which, like the hand, consists of three parts : The tarsus, the metatarsus and the toes. The tarsus consists of seven bones (48–52) ; the metatarsus of five (53, 54), articulating at one extremity with the tarsal bones, and at the other with the first range of toe-bones, and so united as to give the foot a convex form, and conduce to the elasticity of the step. The four smaller toes, like the fingers, have three joints, while the great toe, like the thumb, has two joints.

After this condensed description of the bones we pass on to the muscles, which are of more importance.

CHAPTER II.

THE MUSCLES.

WHO has not been entranced by some melodious, prolonged strain of music, by pearl-like purity of colorature? Who has not been surprised at the sylph-like motions of a *danseuse*, or the grotesque springs of a dancer? And yet few have been conscious wherein lay the mystery of all this. It is, in fact, due to a harmonious action of the muscles. All movements of the human body are made by means of the muscles, which are fastened to the movable bones of the skeleton, and are thrown into action by the nerves.

No harmonious movement is possible without a correct action of the muscles.

We believe, therefore, that it may be said truthfully that a knowledge of the structure and peculiarities of the muscles, of the laws of their training and preservation, is the all-important thing if we would do artistic work, if we would be graceful in our actions in life. The muscles consist of a web of tendons and sinews which possess the capability of contraction and expansion. The contraction of a muscle is followed by a state of relaxation (repose), either voluntarily or resulting from weariness, in which state of repose nourishment is better carried on, as in a state of contraction there is greater consumption of blood and nervous strength.

By gradually-increasing and oft-repeated exercise, by proper nourishment, by a flesh diet, the muscles gain incredibly in size and strength, and obtain their full development, while they are rendered weak and lax by inactivity and the lack of good food.

Gymnasts, dancers and piano-players attest the truth of this as-

THE MUSCLES.

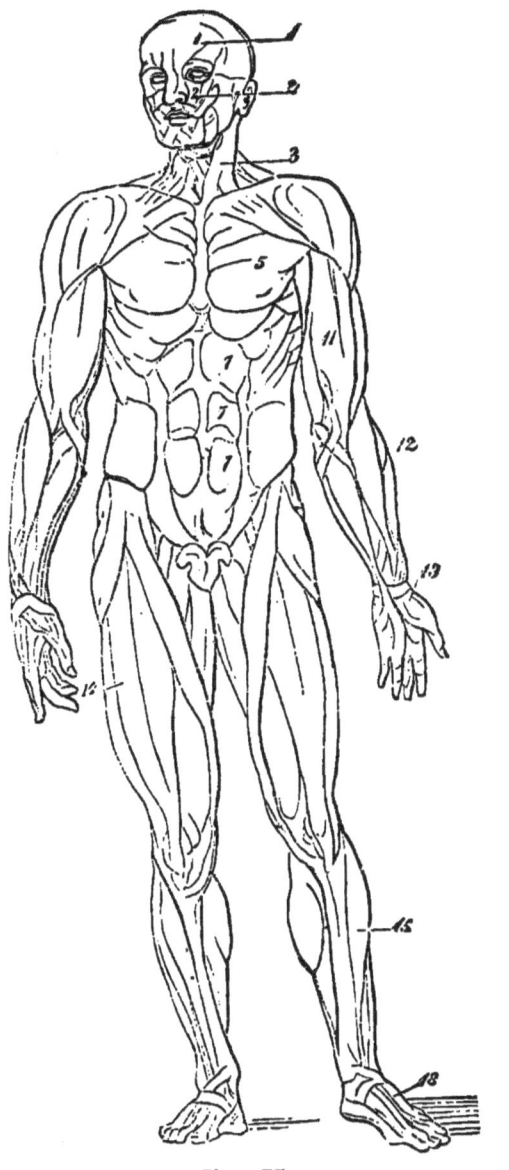

Fig. II.

sertion. Singers, who produce such wonderful effects with those small muscles of the larynx, have brought those muscles to this degree of perfection by the right kind of practice, ever increasing in vigorous effort, and followed by intervals of repose.

As an increased consumption of blood follows contraction of the muscles, so, in the state of repose resulting from the cessation of this contraction, an increased formation of blood takes place; therefore it is self-evident that a muscle acting in steady alternations becomes far stronger, and less easily fatigued, than one whose activity is constant or long continued.

Standing, for this reason, is more fatiguing than walking for the same length of time. Paralysis of the muscles may be brought on by too great or too prolonged exertion. Nothing but a persistent exercise of the muscles, with alternations of the needed repose, will at last fit them to make any movement the will ordains. In the early stages of practice this is impossible, and in the use of certain muscles one cannot guard against moving others with them. Beginners in gymnastics, dancing, fencing, etc., are almost incapable of keeping inactive the muscles that are not required.

The erroneous belief obtains with many that the mind only need be cultivated, and all other culture will follow. But the thought originates in the brain, the brain acts upon the nerves, the nerves upon the muscles, the muscles upon the bones, and only after all these processes is physical action possible. What avails the most intellectual letter if there is no messenger to convey it to the desired place? This is the office of physical gymnastics.

It is only after long practice that the will alone may be relied on to set the required muscles in motion. All who would perform to acceptance before the public, must attain the greatest skill in this respect.

After these brief remarks upon the muscles in general, we proceed to a description of them in detail. They may be divided into two classes., viz., *the voluntary and the involuntary muscles.*

THE MUSCLES.

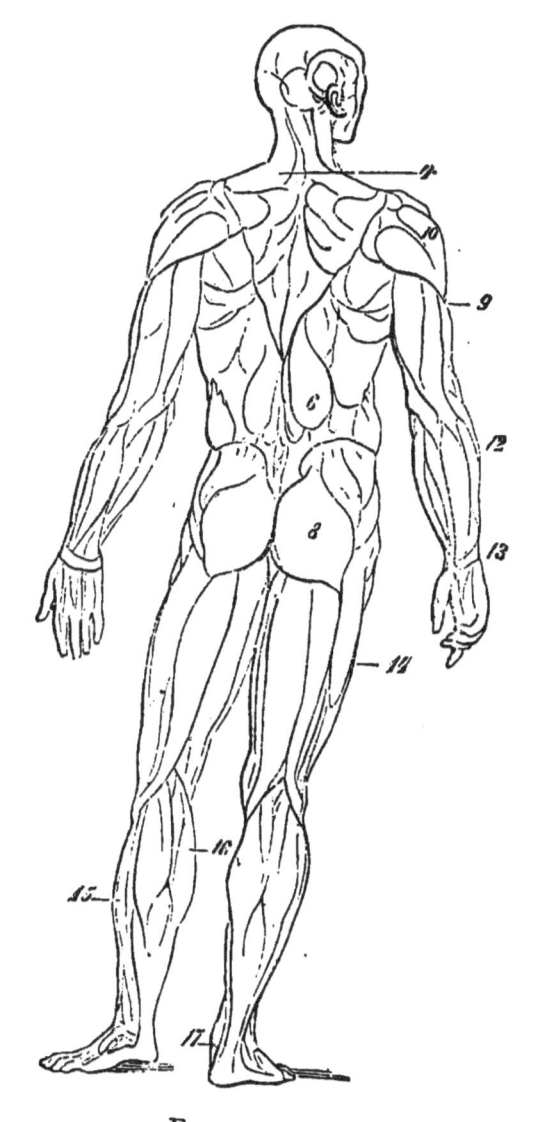

FIG. III.

To the second class belong the *heart*, the *diaphragm*, and the *muscles* of the *intestines*. All the others belong to the first class. We distinguish (*a*) the muscles of the head, (*b*) the muscles of the torso, (*c*) the muscles of the upper limbs, and (*d*) the muscles of the lower limbs.

The Muscles of the Head.

The muscle of the cranium (musculus epicranius), whose front part is called the forehead muscle (musculus frontalis), and has an important part in acting as its office, is to elevate and lower the forehead, as well as to control the eyebrows, and also

The Muscles of the Face.

These, by means of the facial nerve, which controls all these muscles, are closely connected with the brain, and for this reason strong impressions upon the brain, or diseases of that organ, have great influence upon the muscles of the face. They are the means of expressing sensations and passions, and effect the play of the features. Sad and painful emotions generally contract the muscles of the mouth, eyes and forehead, and draw them *downward*. Joyous emotions, into which the cheek muscles also enter, draw them *upward*.

In Figures II. and III. the muscles are designated by numbers as follows :

1. The skull and forehead muscle.
2. The face muscles.
3. The throat muscles.
4. The neck muscles.
5. The chest muscles.
6. The back muscles.
7. The abdominal muscles.
8. The pelvis muscles.
9. The shoulder-blade muscles.
10. The deltoid muscle.
11. The upper-arm muscles.

12. The fore-arm muscles.
13. The hand muscles.
14. The upper-leg muscles.
15. The lower-leg muscles.
16. The muscles of the calf of the leg.
17. The tendon of Achilles.
18. The foot muscles.

The Muscles of the Torso.

These are the muscles of the throat, neck, chest, back, abdomen and pelvis. The throat and neck muscles (Fig. III., 4) move the head forward, backward and sideways, turning and stretching it. The muscles on the inside of the throat, which rule the larynx, demand a special exposition that will not be given here, as it belongs to the domain of singing and rhetoric. The breast muscles (Fig. II., 5), leaving the breastbone uncovered, lie around the whole cavity of the chest, and have the important function of regulating the breathing, as well as moving the shoulders and arms. The muscle which separates the abdominal cavity from that of the chest, performs the main function in breathing, and also serves for contracting the chest-cavity, is called the diaphragm, and must have its special description in the study of singing and speech. The spinal muscles (Fig. III., 6) serve to hold erect, bend and extend the whole torso; they move the shoulders and upper arms, and assist in breathing. The important office of the abdominal muscles is to protect and sustain the organs of the abdomen (intestines). It is to be especially noted that, if these muscles have to perform an arduous work, or to remain a long time in a tense position, they must be contracted, or else injury to the person will result. The abdominal muscles extend from the lower part of the cavity of the chest to the pelvis, and form the front and side walls of the abdomen.

The Muscles of the Upper Limbs.

These may be divided into the following groups : —
1. The muscles of the shoulder extend from the clavicle (col-

lar-bone) and the shoulder-blade to the upper arm, and move it in all directions. The strongest of them is called the deltoid muscle (Fig. III., 10).

2. The muscles of the upper arm (Fig. III., 9, and Fig. II., 11) lie partly upon the inner and partly upon the outer side of the humerus, and serve to bend or stretch the fore-arm.

3. The muscles of the fore-arm (Fig. III., 12) move the hand and fingers inward and outward, bending or stretching, withdrawing or extending them. The hand muscles lie in the hand, especially at the first and fifth joints of the metacarpus (Fig. II., 13).

The Muscles of the Lower Limbs.

These comprise (1) the muscles of the lower leg and foot, and (2) those of the upper leg. The muscles of the upper leg (Fig. III., 14) serve for stretching and bending the knee-joint, and for drawing the leg backward and forward. The tendons, which draw it forward, lie in front; those which draw it backward lie behind. The tendons of the foot and the toes (15) are on the back surface of the lower leg, forming the calf of the leg (Fig. III., 16). They are peculiarly important in walking and dancing. The lower end of the tendon, which is attached to the top of the heel-bone, is called, on account of its strength, the "tendon of Achilles" (Fig. III., 17). The dilating muscles of the foot lie upon its upper surface (Fig. II., 18); those which dilate and contract the toes are in the sole or lower part.

All the mentioned muscles of the first group may be moved voluntarily, and acquire incredible facility through practice. We shall learn in the course of our studies of physical gymnastics how many sorts of these voluntary movements there are.

CHAPTER III.

THE MECHANISM OF THE LIMBS.

THE limbs of the human body move in accordance with the law of the lever. It is not necessary to our purpose to explain this law, and we need offer no further explanation of the arms than that already given in our description of the muscles. It is quite otherwise with the lower limbs, which are governed by special laws relating to the centre of gravity. If these laws are not strictly followed, good walking is impossible. We must, therefore, dwell upon them, first treating of

The Centre of Gravity.

The relations of the centre of gravity to the base, decide whether the body stands or falls. As every single part remains subject to the laws of gravity, it will always be attracted to the earth's centre. If a mass consists of unlike and variously-formed pieces, each of these will, as far as possible, set its gravitating force into action. These opposing influences must, therefore, unite in such a way that their several actions meet at an imaginary point — the centre of gravity. The whole body will then poise itself as if its weight were accumulated at this place. A direct line from this point to the base, therefore, designates its further relations. If this line meets the base, the body stands; if it extends beyond the base, the body falls. All the movements of men and animals obey this law, but the centre of gravity varies with the different positions assumed by the single limbs.

If a grown man lie with his limbs extended in a horizontal position, his arms resting symmetrically upon the lower part of the body, his centre of gravity will be at the region of the last lumbar vertebra. If he sits, the pelvis with its side muscles forms a base proportionally extended. He can then give the upper part of the body a wide range without danger of falling. A too weak or too narrow base involves a loss of equilibrium.

If the man stands still, the outer outlines of the feet form a base inside of which the line of gravity may fall. But there is much less security here than in sitting or lying down. The narrower the base, the more liable one is to fall. For this reason, to stand on tip-toe on a narrow board or rope is unsafe. If one leg

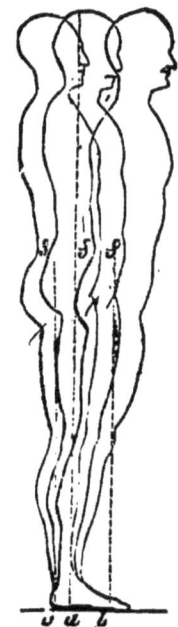

Fig. IV.

swings in the air, this lessens the base, and makes the position more insecure for this and also for other reasons. That part of the body represented by the raised leg, draws the mass to itself, and easily carries it along. One, therefore, instinctively bends the up-

THE MECHANISM OF THE LIMBS.

per part of the body to the opposite side. People with one foot shorter than the other, on this account, often stand obliquely. If a leg is missing, this only adds to the disadvantage, because the centre of gravity is raised higher. Other things being equal, a body rests more firmly the nearer its centre of gravity lies to the base. For this reason, sitting is safer than standing.

If a man stands erect, and with feet close together, the line of gravity falls between the ball of the foot and the heel (Fig. IV., S *a*). If the body bends a little backward, the line of gravity falls at the end of the heel (S *c*). If the body bends forward, it falls between the toes (S *b*). The body standing in a straight line cannot bend beyond these two points without falling.

The line of gravity, as we have just seen, must always fall upon a point of the base on which the body stands; for instance, the man stands erect, with the feet sideways, and a step apart: in this case, the centre of gravity falls right in the middle of the

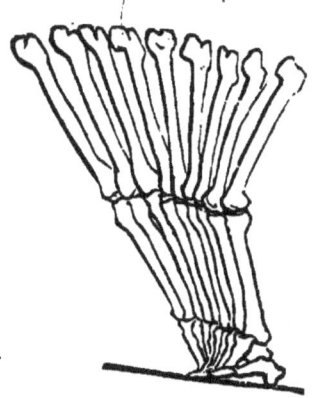

Fig. V.

base on which he stands, equidistant from each foot. If he would now stand upon one leg, this involves a change in tne line of gravity, which is removed to a point under the sole of the foot upon which he stands.

Poses of the body in which the line of gravity is not quite

direct, may be made through various tensions of the muscles, but these are unnatural, awkward and unæsthetic, and should enter into neither the plastic nor the dramatic arts.

The Mechanism of the Walking Apparatus.

Walking depends upon a steady forward movement of the torso over the ground through a periodically repeated action of the legs, which so relieve each other that one alone causes the forward motion, the other, meanwhile, being carried along. The space in which one leg after the other finds itself in this position, embraces exactly two steps. The leg bears the body forward by the tension of one or more of its previously-bent joints (Fig. V.).

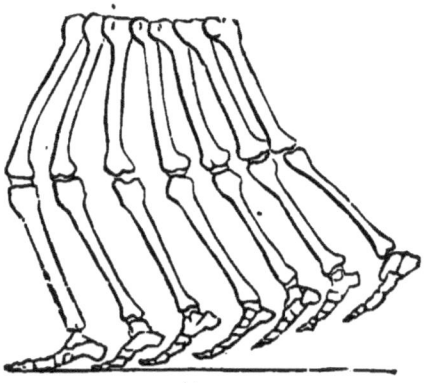

FIG. VI.

The leg that is carried forward while the other remains pendent, swings past the other, carried onward by its own weight alone, around the point of junction with the torso (Fig. VI.). The rapidity of this swinging motion, like that of the pendulum of a clock, depends upon the length of the leg, which also has much influence upon the duration of a step. All persons — children and grown people — move in a tempo proportioned to the length of the legs.

In ordinary walking, the beginning of the extension occurs at the same moment in which the centre point of the socket has just

THE MECHANISM OF THE LIMBS. 19

passed the point of support of the foot. One moment previous, when the one stood vertically over the other, the leg had acquired its utmost limit of flexion (Fig. VII.).

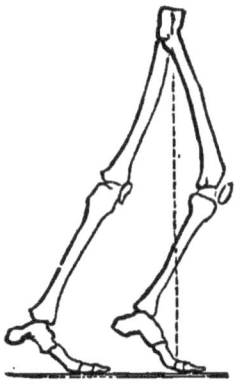

FIG. VII.

The legs, like the other limbs, can be moved forward by the strength of the muscles more rapidly than if impelled by their own weight; but this demands so constant and energetic an exertion of the muscles, that a gait so unnatural cannot long be maintained.

From the moment when the foot is placed in position, and its joints begin to bend, until the moment when the socket of the upper leg stands directly over its point of support, the leg sustains the body through the strength of its muscles without moving it forward; for the other leg can no longer restrain the downward movement of the body caused by its extension. This, therefore, begins the shortening of its motor muscle, through which it not merely secures a descent of the body around the axis of the foot-joint, but at the same time, moves the centre of gravity forward in a more horizontal line (Fig. VIII.).

In the course of this movement the centre of gravity moves forward gradually from the back part of the heel. Until it reaches the ends of the toes, the points of support are successively at other parts of the sole. These move forward in the same manner until the heel is at last raised from the ground, the foot stands upon its toes, and its pendulum-like swinging begins. Meantime the sole is gradually loosed from the ground, and supports itself upon ever new points, like the rim of a carriage wheel rolling over the road (Fig. V.). If, in our usual walking, we compare the periodically-changing activity of one leg, we see, above all, that

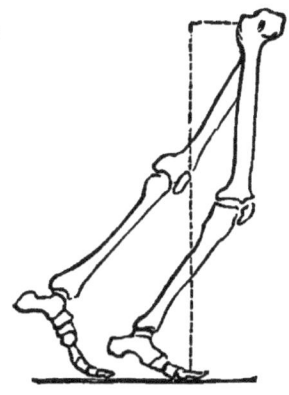

Fig. VIII.

the period the swinging demands is shorter than that in which the leg is occupied, partly in sustaining, partly in moving forward.

As we have said, these two periods of the movements of one leg embrace an interval of two steps. If we seek the parallel movement of both legs inside of this period in the usual gait (Fig. IX.), it is evident that the sustaining leg does not leave the ground at the moment the other begins its swinging by the uplifting of the foot, but somewhat later. Therefore it follows that both feet are for a certain time simultaneously in contact with the ground.

That wavering in the gait, more noticeable in women than in men, owing to the greater breadth of the pelvis in woman, may be remedied by the counter motion of swinging the arms. The drawing forward of the torso by swinging of the legs, may also be

THE MECHANISM OF THE LIMBS.

corrected by swinging the right arm forward with the left leg, and the left arm with the right leg.

The importance of this counter movement of the arms is recognized in the military regulations of the present day, which command absolute freedom of the arms; whereas forty years ago soldierly discipline required that they should be pressed immovably against the sides of the legs.

Hence it follows, that in walking a pendulous movement of the arms should take place. But this must not be too pronounced ; the arms should hang lightly at the sides.

This is the simple mechanism of walking, which is the same in all people having normal organs. The manifold ways of walking depend upon the line of gravity: whether it is moved more slowly

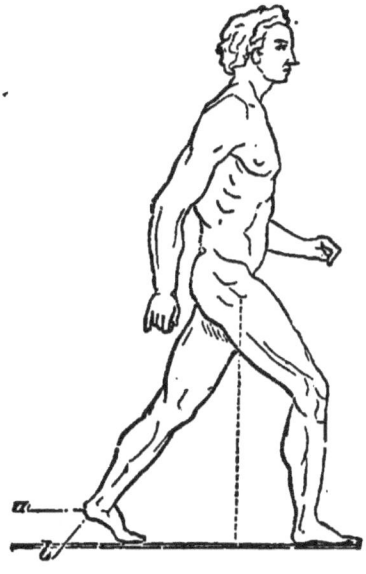

FIG. IX.

or quickly, more regularly or irregularly. The gait also varies with the walking apparatus, with the aim proposed in walking, and is impaired by stiffness, by bad habits, and by affectation.

From all that has been said, it is evident that the natural gait arises, not from strength of muscle (false activity of the muscles), but from the law of gravity. The law of gravity demands that in walking, the body should incline forward. The more rapidly one walks, the more he bends forward. If he inclines forward too much, he must either fall from one foot on to the other, or strain the muscles to prevent falling. If he does not incline forward at all, he moves only by undue exertion of the muscles. We see at a glance whether one moves onward by the law of gravity, or by undue muscular effort.

Walking Forward.

We have now learned the mechanism of simple walking. To recapitulate briefly : —

The leg which is to be thrust forward bends slightly in the knee-socket, and the heel is thus loosed from the floor, while the ball and the toes rest upon it, and the centre of gravity is carried to the other foot. At almost the same moment, the body bends slightly forward, the leg is stretched out ahead, and the foot again plants itself firmly upon the ground. But at the moment when this foot touches the ground, and the centre of gravity is consequently raised, the other foot lifts its heel, and, making a slight pressure upon the ground with ball and toes, moves forward in the same step.

The heel will touch the floor first. This is quite right, but it must be the lower part (Fig. IX., *b*), not the back part (*a*), and no pause must ensue between the setting of the heel and toes upon the ground. This is the simple process of walking, which, however modified, must still retain its main characteristics.

Hence, walking demands three different movements of the legs and feet. First the heel is raised, then the leg is thrust forward, and lastly the foot is set upon the ground, while the other foot lifts its heel, and touches the ground with ball and toes.

To attain security in walking, stated practice is necessary to strengthen the muscles, the gait being quickened gradually.

There is this difference between walking and running: In the former, between every two steps a moment intervenes during which both feet touch the ground ; whilst in the latter this never occurs, both feet, on the contrary, being at times in the air.

Walking Backward

is practiced in this way : — The heel is raised, as in walking forward, the leg is thrust backward, the end of the foot being turned outward with the great toe touching the ground. Then the whole foot is set upon the ground, assuming the centre of gravity, while the other, relieved of the centre of gravity, touches the ground only with the little toe. This foot now passes the stationary foot in a backward direction, and in the same way.

As one proceeds in this practice, he passes from slow to quick, and on to running. This backward step requires much practice as it is used constantly on the stage. It is also in frequent use in court circles and in the *salons* of high life, where a knowledge of it is of great advantage. In walking backward it must be noted that the great toe is first set down with the knee bent very much outward, and that it is not the flat sole or the heel which first touches the floor. From the latter cause arise the awkward backward movements of untrained people. A tyro, in stepping backward, is sure to let his heel first touch the floor.

So much in regard to the mechanism of walking. We shall treat in "Æsthetic Gymnastics" of walking as indicative of character and passion, of walking as produced by habit and by affectation.

PART SECOND.

PHYSICAL GYMNASTICS.

"The Greeks first made themselves into beautiful forms, before they expressed such objects in marble and painting."

HEGEL'S "Philosophy of History."

INTRODUCTION TO PART SECOND.

Our foregoing observations in regard to things necessary for the pupil to know at the outset, lead us next to that practice which strengthens his muscles and ensures him the use of his limbs, so that they may later become æsthetically serviceable to his will.

We would not have single muscles stimulated through practice to unusual strength, or to the capability of producing masterpieces. We demand that all the muscles, the least as well as the greatest, should receive that training which is indispensable to easy, graceful movements, and we have, therefore, selected such exercises as may be undertaken in any place, and without preparation or apparatus. We have not sought to include all those exercises supposed to belong to the rubric of physical gymnastics, but have laid aside all machine practice. Our book is not for children, but for grown people who would pursue what they neglected in youth, or what unfavorable circumstances denied them. The author is certain, however, that this system answers the purpose, and leads to the desired end, he having tested it by years of application in his own teaching.

DIRECTIONS FOR PRACTICE.

Those who would pursue this practice of gymnastics without injury, and with benefit to the health, must strictly follow the directions here briefly laid down : —

1. The most suitable time for practice is shortly before breakfast, dinner or supper. The best time is in the morning before breakfast. After exercise, a pause of half, or at least a quarter of an hour must ensue before eating, as digestion cannot be well

carried on in an excited state of the muscles. No exercise must be taken upon a full stomach.

2. Success results only from perseverance. If the desired end is to be reached, practice must be carried on with great regularity.

3. Before beginning, all oppressive clothing must be removed; neck, chest and abdomen must be free from pressure. Women must remove every sort of corset.

4. If, during practice, a decided rush of blood to the head is remarked, or a quickened pulsation of the heart with rapid breathing, the exercise must be carried on very circumspectly and moderately, with long pauses; that is, between every two exercises there must be a normal action of the lungs.

5. During exercise, the breath must not be held in. On the contrary, draw the air slowly, and in deep draughts, into the lungs, and expel it just as slowly, not forgetting to contract the abdominal muscles.

A right action of the lungs is indispensable for the preservation of man, since upon this depend the soundness of the lungs, the proper circulation of the blood, and the health of the whole body.

The pauses between the exercises are, therefore, used for deep breathing, which is practiced by inhaling the air slowly, and in as great quantities as possible, and expelling it just as slowly.

Diseases of all sorts result, in great measure, from defective breathing, as very many, and hysterical persons in particular, breathe only with the upper half of the lungs, thus injuring the lower half through lack of expansion. This frequently leads to consumption in youth, and to asthma in old age.

6. The movements must be slow, but decided and energetic.

It is well in exercising to observe a certain measure, with counts either loud or silent, which may cease as perfection is acquired by practice.

In the beginning make an exercise five to eight times; after a few days, ten to fifteen times; after three or four weeks, twenty to thirty times. Never repeat an exercise oftener.

Above all, guard against entire fatigue of the muscles. As soon as an undue sense of weariness comes on, the exercise must be stopped or deferred until it is over. Be content with small results at first. Strength and ease will come with practice.

That disagreeable tension of the muscles which ensues at first, need not cause alarm in regard to the health, and induce one to abandon gymnastic practice. Injury results only from senseless over-excitation of the muscles. A gradual progress in exercise should be observed ; a safe and steady passage from easy to difficult things.

7. Exercise must be carried on in pure air. If within doors, the place should be thoroughly ventilated by opening doors and windows before the practice begins. It must not be prosecuted in jerks and starts. Women should be exceedingly careful in this regard.

The double organs (arms, hands, legs, shoulders and hips) should be exercised right and left alternately.

CHAPTER I.

THE SINGLE MEMBERS — SIMPLE EXERCISES.

Base Position.

THE exercise begins with knees outstretched, heels close together, toes turned outward so that the soles of both feet form the sides of a right angle, the chest moderately expanded, the

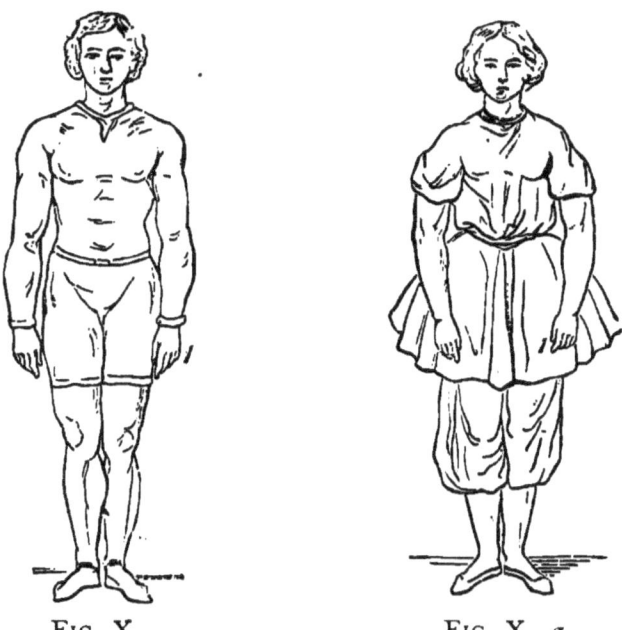

FIG. X. FIG. X., *a*.

shoulders thrown back, the hands hanging lightly at the sides or resting upon the hips, and a perfectly erect attitude. This position we call the *base position* (Figs. X. and X., *a*).

THE SINGLE MEMBERS.

HEAD AND NECK EXERCISES.

Turning the Head to the Right and Left.

The head is turned slowly to the right without lowering it, as far as the muscles of the neck allow (Fig. XI.). Remaining

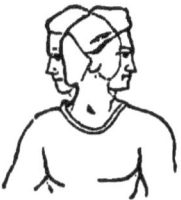

FIG. XI.

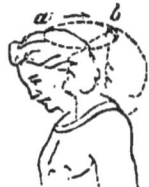

FIG. XII.

some time in this position greatly strengthens the muscles of the throat and neck. The same practice is then observed by turning the head to the left, while the body remains in its *base position*, and the shoulder-muscles are motionless.

The object of this practice is to give freedom to the muscles of the neck. This is very necessary, for in gesture it constantly occurs, notably in persons of high rank, that a slight turn of the head to one side or the other, without the least movement of the body, is of great significance. When, through inflexibility of the muscles of the neck, arising from want of exercise, the whole body turns with it, as we often observe in persons without gymnastic training, the effect is very ungraceful.

Bowing of the Head Forward, Backward, or to the Right and Left.

The head is bowed in a fourfold way, the trunk remaining erect, without stretching the neck-muscles too powerfully.

The backward inclination of the neck, especially in women, should be slight (Fig. XII.).

From this fourfold exercise of the head proceeds one exercise : —

The Head Circle.

The four head movements are united by a circular line (Fig. XII., *a–b*), and also make a funnel-shaped movement without the passing of the head to its normal position. From the forward inclination of the head we pass to the backward movements back on the left and right sides, then again to the first forward movement, the upper part of the body remaining in its *base position*, and the uninterrupted circular form slightly indicated.

A strong, muscular neck is not a feminine trait surely; but women often greatly strengthen the muscles of the head and neck by gymnastic exercises. While the neck has to sustain the not inconsiderable weight of the head, an oblique carriage of the head may be easily brought on if the neck, from weakness or relaxation of its muscles, cannot perform the required service. In case of this oblique carriage of the head, mothers and teachers have sometimes used collars set with bristles so arranged that the bristles at once cause a disagreeable sensation if the neck inclines to one side. Tissot tells of the superior of a convent who corrected this habit by instituting a sort of game in which a ball or some other slippery object was carried on the head, the pupil who let it fall paying a forfeit.

A lady pupil came to the author of this work, — a singer who after two years' study with another teacher, could not sing a note without turning her head considerably toward the right shoulder, which, while giving her an awkward appearance, also greatly injured the tone. He adopted the following method: As soon as she began to sing he had her turn her head to the left shoulder, not allowing her to sing a note in any other position. After some months when he saw that the inclination to the right shoulder had wholly disappeared, he let her hold her head erect. Now in singing there was a conflict between the right and left muscles, but the effort to obey neither much facilitated the erect position of the head, and the oblique leaning was wholly cured.

TORSO EXERCISES.

Shoulder Movements.

Both shoulders are raised as high and as forcibly as possible

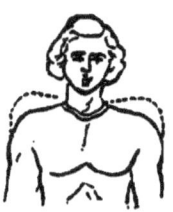

Fig. XIII.

THE SINGLE MEMBERS.

(Fig. XIII.), and then allowed to fall slowly into their normal position. A too rapid fall will shake the head too much.

This exercise is first performed with both shoulders, and then with one, the *base position* being strictly observed, even in regard to the arms, which must fall loosely down from the shoulders, without bending the elbows. The shoulders are then drawn forward and backward, first singly and then both together. From this movement results

The Shoulder Circle.

A movement upward, backward, and downward, forward and again upward (without interruption), not by jerks, but in a circle.

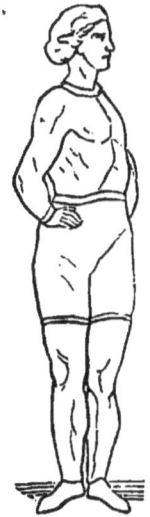

FIG. XIV.

The same movement may be made in a reversed order with the shoulders elevated, forward, downward, backward, upward, etc.

In all practice only the required muscles should be active, all the others being in perfect repose. This rule is to be strictly observed.

Rising and Falling of the Hips.

The leg fully extended is drawn by means of the hips up toward the torso, and then allowed to fall slowly.

This movement is much restricted, as the foot cannot be raised more than two or three finger breadths from the floor.

The Turning or Twisting of the Trunk.

The trunk is turned to the right or left with the legs extended in a straight line, as if it would turn around on its own axis without moving the hips (Fig. XIV.). This movement is limited, but it is beneficial to the abdomen and to the lower muscles of the back and hips.

Inclination of the Torso Forward, Backward, Right and Left.

The legs are extended, the torso from the hips to the skull bending forward until the torso and legs form a right angle (Fig. XV.), then they pass slowly back to the *base position*. This

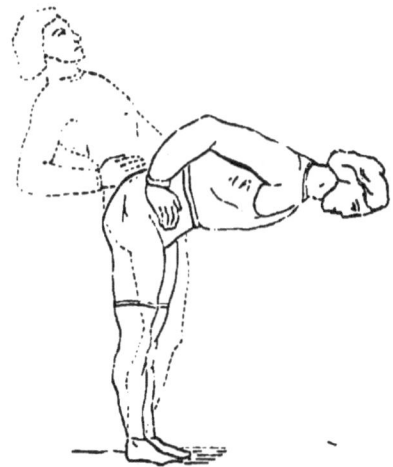

Fig. XV.

exercise, slow at first, grows more rapid until at last it assumes a sort of violence, as if the upper part of the body were thrown to the earth, and must be raised forcibly.

THE SINGLE MEMBERS.

The side movements (Fig. XVI.), and especially the backward movement (Fig. XV.) can be executed only in a restrictive way. From the exercises just described arises

The Torso Circle,

which is formed in the same manner as the head circle (Fig. XVI, *a, b, c*.). But here no revolution on the axis takes place, as the front of the torso must always retain the same position.

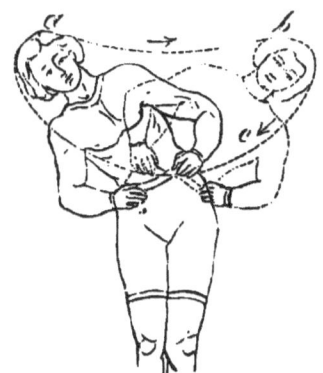

Fig. XVI.

This exercise is most easily practiced with the hands at the hips (akimbo). It gives excellent training to the muscles of the back and abdomen, an indispensable requisite in speaking and singing, as well as in every position requiring great effort. It must be performed at the last with much energy of movement.

Elevating the Torso.

The pupil lies horizontally upon the back with limbs extended, hands crossed over the breast or falling at the sides, and without changing the position of the limbs or separating the feet, which must touch each other at the heels, slowly and gently rises to a sitting posture, and then lies down again.

Some pupils will find it impossible to go through with this exercise at first. In this case, as well as in that of persons with weak abdominal muscles, a pillow is placed under the head, or they grasp some fixed object with the toes in order to maintain the equilibrium. After a while these aids can be dispensed with. The object of this exercise is to strengthen the abdominal muscles.

Torso exercises, that is, an activity of the muscles of the back, have an invigorating influence upon the spinal marrow, and are all the more beneficial because exercise of the muscles of the back is greatly neglected in every-day life.

All these exercises should be pursued with great industry, and, above all others, those pertaining to the shoulders. Nothing can be more stiff, awkward and ungainly than a shrug of the shoulders in which the whole torso moves. To ladies, especially, ease in the shoulder-movements is indispensable.

To quote the words of Dr. Kloss, in his "Home Gymnastics for Women:" — "When one reflects what influence the shoulders have in the development of the bust, those exercises, which prevent a muscular laxness in this region, should be prized as a means of beauty if the strengthening of the shoulder-muscles had not a greater significance as a means for promoting health. Any injurious pressure upon the shoulders must be transferred to the region of the chest that lies beneath them."

Arm Exercises.

The action of the arms and hands is of great importance in acting and in gesture, because, next to the face, they are most capable of expression. Special attention must, therefore, be given

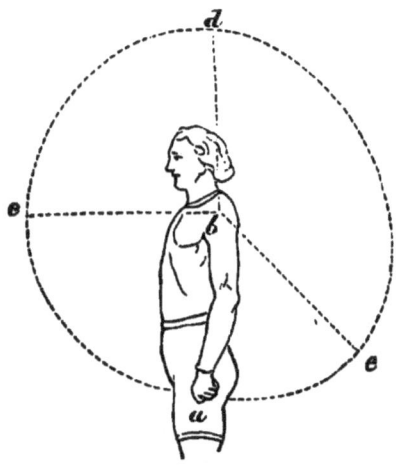

FIG. XVII.

to the training of these muscles, and to the easy movement of their joints. The wrist-joint is of great importance in gesture, and much effort must be applied to rendering the hand free from the lower arm.

ARM EXERCISES WITH OUTSTRETCHED ARMS.

1. Lifting and Moving the Arm.

The arm is lifted and extended slowly forward and upward (Fig. XVII., *a, c, d*), and then, with a slight swing, allowed to fall back into the base position and beyond it (*a–e*). Both these movements are slow at first, but grow more rapid until swinging. The hand is left open, or it is clinched. The backward movement is a limited one.

Lifting the Arm. — This is done sideways while the extended arm is raised in a lateral direction, first with the outer and then with the inner palm of the hand upward, until it touches the side of the head, when it falls back to the base position. Here, also, the full swing is made gradually.

When, by means of the foregoing exercises, the pupil has attained perfect mastery over his shoulder-joints, he passes over to

2. The Arm Circle.

This is made as follows : — The arm being lifted as described in section 1, is passed forward and backward, and *vice versa*, until it resumes the base position, as in Fig. XVII., *a, c, d, e–a.* The movement begins slowly, growing more rapid until it is a swinging movement. It is more elliptical than circular, but, by frequent practice, can be made to approach very nearly to a circular form.

The shoulder-muscles, and those around the cavity of the chest, are set into action by these movements, whose main object is to impart freedom to the shoulder-joint and to strengthen respiration, which is greatly facilitated by the expansion of the chest.

3. Turning and Revolving the Arms.

The extended arm is raised sideways to the height of the shoulder, so that the outer palm of the hand is uppermost; the

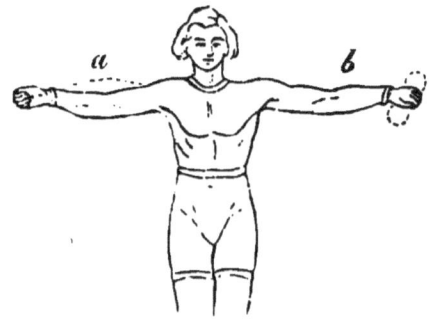

Fig. XVIII.

inner palm is then turned upward, and this is done alternately, with the wrist-joint as stiff as possible. The same exercise is then carried on with the hand clinched (Fig. XVIII., *a*).

This movement will be most perfectly executed if the pupil imagines himself driving a gimlet into a piece of wood with his outstretched arm.

4. *Balancing and Oblique Movements.*

The outstretched arms are moved forward (See Fig. LXVIII., *a, d–a*) so that the inner palms meet, and then backward as if

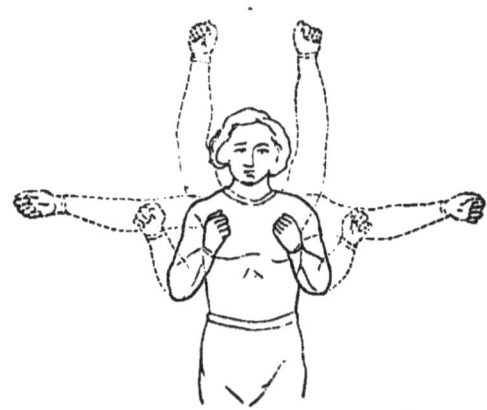

Fig. XIX.

THE SINGLE MEMBERS. 39

they would meet behind the back, which they cannot do wholly. This movement begins slowly, growing more rapid until swinging is attained. The oblique movement consists in raising the arm, not to the height of the shoulder, but to that of the elbow (See Fig. LXVIII., *a*, *c–d*), and is executed in the same manner. In this way the outer palms of the hands can be carried behind the back until they touch, especially by rapid, powerful swinging. In both these movements the front muscles of the chest act alternately, half the front and half the back wall of the chest-cavity acting in unison. They facilitate breathing.

ARM EXERCISES WITH THE AID OF THE ELBOW-JOINTS.

The movements of the elbow-joint are of a twofold sort — the flexor and the extensor movements, or the attraction and repulsion of the lower arm from the upper arm.

1. Attraction and Repulsion.

This happens when the lower arms are drawn upward from the base position until the clinched hands nearly touch the shoulders. The lower arm is then allowed to fall tense with strained mus-

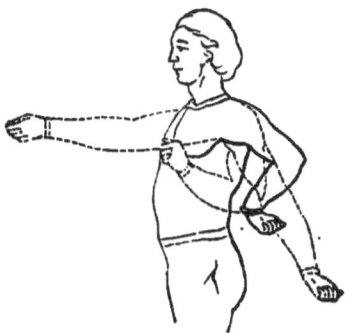

FIG. XX.

cles, even with a sort of thrust, back to the base position. This exercise can be carried out downward, upward, forward, outward and backward, in a limited degree (See Figs. XIX. and XX.).

40 ÆSTHETIC PHYSICAL CULTURE.

During the downward movement the upper arms remain in the base position; in all other sorts of repulsion they are obliged to follow the lower arm. In regard to the foot, it may be remarked that the centre of gravity rests more upon the toes than upon the heel, in order to avoid too great concussion of the brain.

If the fore part of the hand is now placed upon the shoulder, the movement is made from the elbow, as if one would strike out from behind (eight or ten times), an excellent exercise for expanding the chest.

2. *Movement of the Arms Behind the Back.*

The hands are folded behind the back near the loins, so that the inner palms join; then the pupil seeks to extend the arms without loosening the hands, raising, as far as possible, the arms

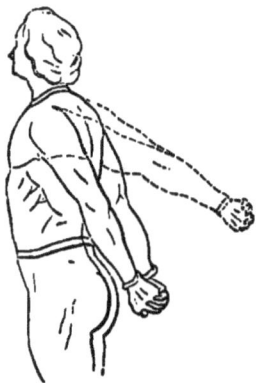

Fig. XXI.

still extended stiffly behind (Fig. XXI.), lets them down again, and goes on thus, slowly at first, and then more rapidly. The spine must not be bent.

By these movements the shoulders are tensely and strongly drawn back, the extension drawing them downward and thus enforcing a bearing noble and conducive to health, while the front wall of the chest is widened and breathing facilitated. They are a safe-guard against protrusion of the shoulders, against

THE SINGLE MEMBERS. 41

laxness and paralysis of the back shoulder-muscles, which may be discerned in a crooked posture of the body and an inability to correct it by an effort of the will; they also prevent most sorts of chronic asthma.

HAND AND WRIST PRACTICE.

The arms and hands extended sideways are brought into equilibrium (with the outer palms upward). The hands are now raised by a mere wrist-movement, the fingers remaining stiff, and carried upward, downward, forward, backward and in a circle, the outstretched arm still retaining its position. Each of these exercises is practiced six times. Then the fingers are closed upon the palm, and the several movements, just described, are again made, assuming gradually the form of a perpendicular figure 8, and at last that of a horizontal one (∞).

Finger-Stretching and Spreading.

This exercise is accompanied by that of spreading and stretching the fingers, the clinched hand being opened suddenly as if something were thrown violently away. Then the fingers are

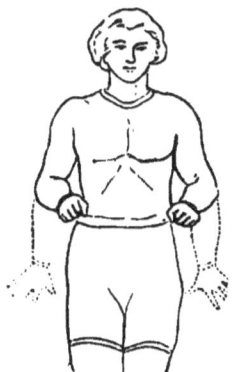

FIG. XXII.

spread as widely as possible, and this again, as if they had to overcome some opposition with muscles tensely drawn, claw-like, and contracted to a fist. This practice is carried out with arms pendent, the lower arm being drawn slightly toward the upper one, and then thrust away, the fingers being spread suddenly (Fig. XXII.).

Unimportant as these exercises may seem, they give freedom to the wrist-joint, which can be acquired in no other way, and the importance of this joint in gesture is universally known. If the wrist is stiff, an arm-movement will be awkward and angular; but with a stiff elbow and a flexible wrist, the movement can be tolerated. Even the movement of a finger is of the greatest importance in gesture, but the first rule is to be sparing of movements of the hands and fingers.

Graceful movements of hand and fingers are of very great importance to women, on account of delicate, feminine handiwork, as well as fine and graceful gestures.

LEG AND FOOT PRACTICE.

1. Exercise with Stretched Leg — Leg Swinging.

The tense leg is raised somewhat from the floor, then gradually as far as possible, and the pupil stands for a long time upon

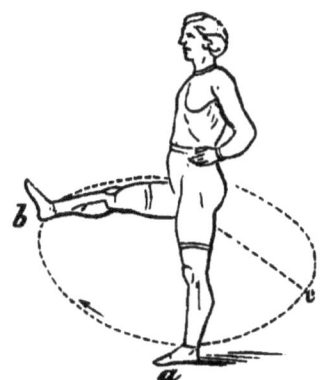

FIG. XXIII.

one leg (Fig. XXIII., *a, b*). Then the leg is going backward (*a, c*), then sideways in the same manner, until the full swing is completed. From these movements arises

THE SINGLE MEMBERS.   43

2. *The Leg Circle, Forward and Backward*,
as represented in Fig. XXIII., *a, b, c, a,* a circle having more or less the elliptical form, and then backward, *a, c, b, a*.

MOVEMENT OF THE HIP AND KNEE-JOINTS.

1. The Flexion and Extension of the Knee Backward.

The lower leg passes backward, the upper leg standing still, until both form a right angle; first slowly, and then more rapidly; then on until the lower leg passes over the line of the right angle with the heel almost touching the breech (Fig. XXIV., *b*). The centre of gravity rests at the point of the stationary foot, to avoid jarring the brain. This exercise, if performed rapidly, is attended with a sort of swing. Then the knee still remaining tense, the leg is thrown with some violence back into the base position without striking upon the floor.

2. The Flexion and Extension of the Knee Forward.

The upper leg is thrown forward, the lower leg falling perpendicularly so that both form a right angle (Fig. XXIV., *c, d*);

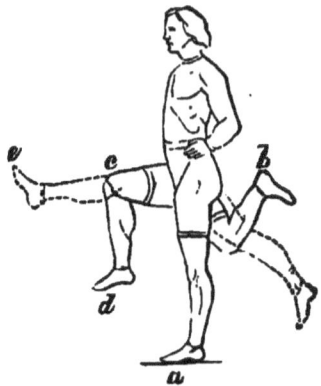

FIG. XXIV.

then the lower leg is extended slowly so that it is at length in equilibrium, and forms a right angle with the stationary leg (*a*, *e*). It then passes slowly back to the base position. After some practice this is done with facility.

The object of this exercise is to strengthen the flexor and extensor muscles of the knee, and give freedom to the knee-joint. Exercises with a like purpose, and which the author has seen attended with beneficial results to his own pupils, are also introduced into his system. He calls them simply exercises for

3. Strengthening the Muscles of the Leg.

I.

(*a*) The right leg takes a long stride out of the base position (farther than in Fig. LXVII.), while the sole of the left foot remains fixed upon the floor. The hands are then braced against the hips, and the upper part of the body, held in a vertical position, with chest expanded and shoulders thrown back, is allowed to sink toward the knee of the right leg, while the left leg remains stiff. The natural result is that the right knee passes beyond the line of the toes. When the utmost limits of the flexion are reached, the body remains for a short time in this position; then (*b*) without raising the sole of either foot from the floor, the body is allowed to sink toward the knee of the left leg, the right leg being held stiff, and to remain as long a time as before. Then (*c*) a full swaying of the upper part of the body takes place (from *a* to *b* and *vice versa*), increasing in rapidity until the swing is complete. This exercise is performed ten or twelve times.

II.

The exercise given under I., *a*, is carried out, and when the forward knee has reached the utmost limit of tension, the centre of gravity is carried over to this leg alone, while the stationary leg is raised from the floor, so that the pupil stands upon one strongly bent leg, while the other is thrust stiffly backward into the air. This position is retained a long time, then the same movement is repeated with the other leg.

III.

Exercise II. is practiced with the leg extended and bent alternately ten or twelve times in rapid succession, so that the upper

THE SINGLE MEMBERS. 45

part of the body, still held in a strictly vertical position, sinks and rises by turns.

These exercises are excellent. They impart strength to the knee-joint, making kneeling and rising far more easy, adding firmness to the gait, and improving the carriage of the whole body.

MOVEMENT OF THE HIP, KNEE AND FOOT-JOINTS.

1. Foot-Extension.

(*a.*) The pupil rises slowly from the base position, his hands resting against the hips, his heels close together, and sinks downward just as slowly, standing for a long time upon the toes; then ever more rapidly without touching the floor with his heels, he

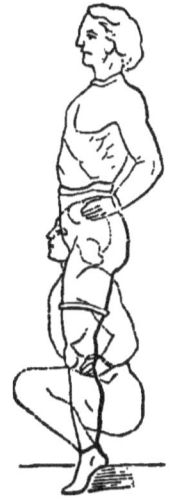

FIG. XXV.

steps briskly up and down; (*b*) then standing upon the toes, he sinks slowly and with closed knees into a sitting posture, remaining in it for some time; then (*c*) into a cowering posture of some duration (Fig. XXV.); then (*d*) he again rises to a sitting posture retaining it for some time, then passes back to the base position without having separated his heels during this whole interval. At last (*e*) he condenses exercises (*b*, *c*) and (*d*) into one, passing from the base position to (*b*), (*c*) and (*d*), and without pause, returning to it again. This last exercise goes on from eight to ten times without interruption. Throughout all the gradations of this practice, the upper part of the body must remain strictly vertical.

This exercise gives freedom to the muscles of the legs and feet. As it requires great effort, it is practiced only a few times in succession, until the muscles have become perceptibly strengthened.

2. *Foot Extension, Flexion and Circling*.

The foot is raised, the knee stretched, being somewhat thrown forward, the toes against the floor and turned outward. They are then drawn upward toward the knee, and then downward six or ten times; then to one side and then the other. From these movements results the foot circle (necessarily very limited; Fig. XXVI.).

The shin-bone, the muscles of the calf of the leg, in fact all the muscles of the lower leg are thus brought into action. This movement serves to give freedom to the ankle-joint, the tarsus and the toes.

Everyone who, without gymnastic training, appears in public and feels as if his feet were filled with lead and his legs were iron bars, recognizes how important it is to give strength and elasticity to these muscles.

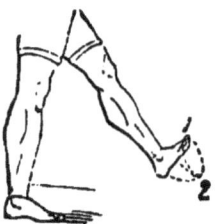

Fig. XXVI.

CHAPTER II.

THE LIMBS AS A WHOLE — COMPLEX EXERCISES.

The object of the exercises given thus far, has been to develop certain muscles singly; those we now give will set all the muscles in action simultaneously to a greater or less degree, and are, to a certain extent, the result of all the preceding exercises.

If the student has diligently practiced the exercises hitherto given, he need not go through them all daily; but he must practice those we now give every morning, if he would have his limbs remain supple and his movements graceful.

The great singer Mme. Schröder-Devrient, whom the world looked upon as one of those favored geniuses, to whom everything comes in sleep, once said to the author of this work: "While I remained upon the stage, and this was quite a long time, I went through certain gymnastic practices every morning. They at length became indispensable to me, and to-day, as an elderly woman, I still continue them."

The oft-repeated maxim, "Everything comes to genius over night," is belied by this assertion of one of the greatest of geniuses.

1. Exercises for the Upper Part of the Body.

(*a*) Begin with the following movements: The hands should be brought from the base position (in which the arms hang loosely at the sides) toward each other, in front of the body, until the index fingers nearly touch (Fig. XXVII., 1, 2). Then raise the arms above the head with a round, graceful movement on the dotted line from 2 to 3. Let them remain in this position some time, describing a half-circle, the tips of the index fingers almost meeting; then loose the circle gradually, letting both arms fall slowly back to the base position at the side (3, 4, 5, 6, 1).

This exercise should be performed at first slowly, accompanied by slow, deep breathing. The chest is dilated, and the move-

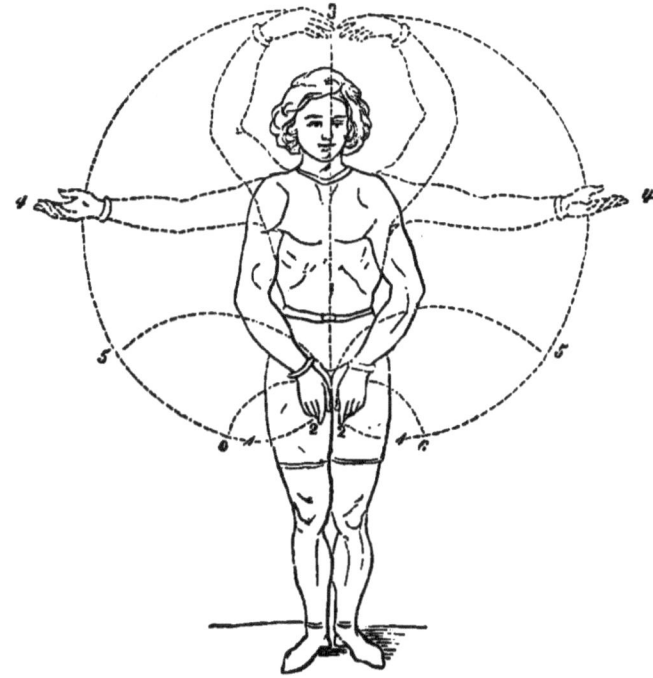

Fig. XXVII.

ments should be made faster and faster up to a regular swinging of the arms.

Breathing from the lower part of the chest, as prescribed for speaking and singing, must, of course, be practiced here; for, when the arms are raised above the head, the upper muscles of the chest are at their highest elevation, and the lower cavity of the chest must expand.

This exercise is the first in our system which demands more

than a mere bending and stretching of the limbs. It forms the basis of the *port de bras* of the art of dancing. Like all the complex exercises which follow, it must have an element of grace. The upper arms should begin the movement, which must be at once visible in the entire arm, even to the finger-tips. Moving the lower arm first, produces angularity and stiffness. We shall come, further on, to the fundamental rules for arm-movements, which will be treated at some length.

The hands must follow easily and gracefully the movements of the lower arm, the palms being somewhat narrowed unless it is absolutely necessary to spread them, as in a repellent movement.

(*b*) Perform exercise (*a*) with one arm at a time, the other hanging gracefully at the side.

(*c*) Perform exercise (*a*) raising the arms only to the height of the shoulders, and when the arms, in returning to the base position, are stretched out on a level with the shoulders. Retain them for a time horizontally extended (Fig. XXVII., 4-4), and then let them sink into the base position.

(*d*) Perform exercise (*a*) without extending the movement above the level of the hips, first with both arms, and then with one at a time (5-5).

(*e*) Perform exercise (*a*) in such a way that the principal movement shall proceed from the wrist, and to a slight extent from the elbow-joint (1, 2, 6, 1).

(*f*) Perform exercise (*a*) turning the trunk to the left until the arms stand over the head (3). Retain this position for a time with the look directed upward, and then complete the exercise while the trunk is being brought back to the base position; then, without any pause, repeat the same exercise, turning the trunk to the right. Continue with this alternating exercise for some time, gradually increasing the rapidity of the movements and keeping the head and look as above mentioned.

The exercises (*b*), (*c*) and (*d*) should then be practised in the same manner; first with both arms, then with one.

2. *Exercises for the Legs and Feet — The "Leg Circle."*

(*a*) One leg is bent slightly at the knee-joint at "1," as in walking forward, the heel being raised from the ground, and the

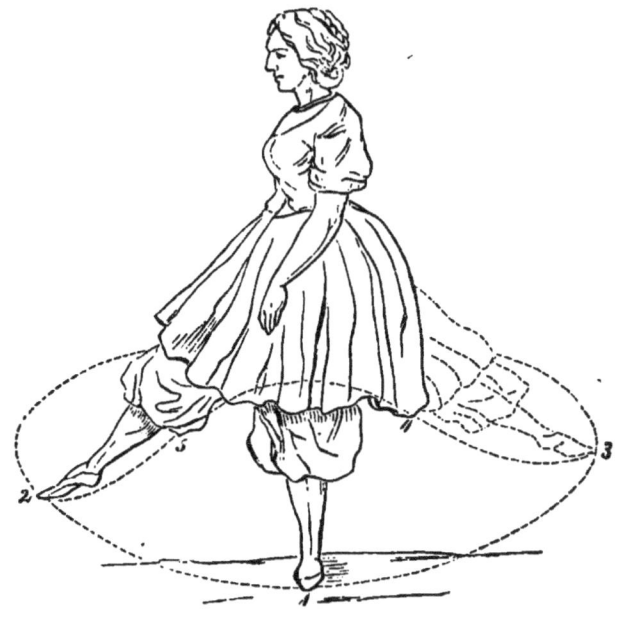

FIG. XXVIII.

centre of gravity transferred to the other foot. At "2," this leg is lifted as high as possible, the toes being turned outward; at "3" it is moved sideways and backward (Fig. XXVIII., 3), describing three-fourths of an ellipse; at "4" the knee is bent, the toes being turned outward and downward, and the heel drawn upward, and the leg is brought past the stationary leg and then extended again forward, this last movement being performed with a certain stress. The base position having been resumed, the same exercise should be immediately performed with the other leg.

(*b*) Repeat exercise (*a*) a number of times, gradually reducing the elevation of the leg and the size of the circle, until at last the movements are performed with the lower leg, and finally with the foot alone.

3. *Exercises for the Upper Body, Legs and Feet.*

(*a*) The exercises given in sections 1 and 2, *a*, should be taken together. First with both arms and one foot; then with one arm and one foot, the right foot and the left arm, and vice versa.

(*b*) Perform the exercises in sections 1 and 2, *a*, up to the point at which the foot is carried farthest backward, and then remain for a time standing on one leg, the hands held lightly over the head, the upper portion of the body much bent forward, and the look turned upward; and from time to time making a flexor and extensor movement with the stationary leg — first slowly, then more rapidly. Then, bending the body backward, bring the foot forward (Fig. XXVIII., as is shown by the dotted line 3, 4, 5, 2), the toes directed downward and outward; at the same moment place the arms in the position shown in Figure XXVII., 4, 4, and make again the flexor and extensor movements with the stationary leg.

This movement of the legs forward and backward, with the corresponding arm movements, should be performed several times in succession, and with each change the flexor and extensor movements should be made six or eight times in quick succession.

(*c*) Walk forward and backward according to the rules given for walking, counting, as you go, one, two, three, keeping the arms above the head, and with each step remain for a short time resting firmly on one leg, while the other is held backward in the air or forward in walking backward.

(*d*) Walk, according to the rules, forward and backward, counting as before, but without stopping at each step, and perform without interruption the exercises with the arms, 1, 2, 3, 4, etc. (as in Fig. XXVII.). The arms must not pass abruptly from one number to the other, but gracefully describe a circle.

The exercises under (*c*) and (*d*), the latter first with one arm, and then with both, should be performed for five minutes.

All these movements must be made exactly in the designated order, and practiced every morning during one's life-time by artists, whether men or women, if they would keep their limbs supple.

Some of the dancing steps will be of great value to the pupil. These steps, under their well-known French names, are as follows:

1. *Les petits battements.*
2. *Changement des pieds.*
3. *Port de bras.*
4. *Pas de basque.*

They will be fully described hereafter.

Instruction in Physical Gymnastics, so far as is necessary to our system, is now ended, and we proceed to Æsthetic Gymnastics and the principles of acting.

Only by a thorough study of Physical Gymnastics, can the pupil become capable of practicing Æsthetic Gymnastics.

PART THIRD.

ÆSTHETIC GYMNASTICS.

INTRODUCTION TO PART THIRD.

THE office of æsthetic gymnastics is to unite in a harmonious whole the limbs of the human body, which have been strengthened and rendered elastic by physical gymnastics; to regulate their movements by the fixed laws of beauty, so that the emotions of the soul may be clearly and beautifully expressed.

This portion of our work comprises two divisions: (1) The pure plastic and universally beautiful, which embraces the subjective of men in real life; and (2) the play of mien and gesture, or the objective, which appears upon the stage in the delineation of other men. We call the first part the Plastic, and the second part the Mimic.

By plastic we understand not repose alone, but also the transition from repose to movement, and from one position to another; that is, beauty in movement, or the "animated plastic."

CHAPTER I.

THE PLASTIC.

1. Of the Human Body and its Limbs.

Standing.—The posture must be in no way stiff, forced or artificial, but free and unrestrained. The body, from crown to sole, must form a perpendicular line (women may incline the head slightly forward); the line of gravity, whether the feet be in contact or separated, passing as nearly as possible through the centre of the base. If the line of gravity falls toward either end of the base, that is, if the body rests too much on one leg, these disadvantages ensue: The body, by reason of a slight weariness, is forced to sustain itself, first on one leg and then on the other, and thus mar every impression of decorum or grace; the hip, on the side on which the body rests, will protrude and produce an awkward appearance; the upper part of the body is also thrown out of the vertical line, and the shoulders, in the movements of the arms, will form oblique lines. The most convenient, and, at the same time, most agreeable position, is that designated in dancing as the fourth, in which that foot is placed forward which is on the side of the person addressed. The foremost foot must always stand next to the interlocutor (Fig. XXIX., *a*). Sustaining the body on this foot, and setting forward the other, is the mark of an awkward person.

In all our elucidations we refer only to persons in cultured circles. If the actor has to personate those in other spheres, he must take lessons from life in its manifold gradations, omitting, of course, everything that positively offends the æsthetic sense.

2. The Limbs Singly, in a State of Rest.

Let the head rest lightly and gracefully upon the neck, held perpendicularly, the chin being in a horizontal position, and the eyes avoiding a fixed upward or downward look. Let the mouth remain closed, but not with compressed lips, and breathing take place through the nose.

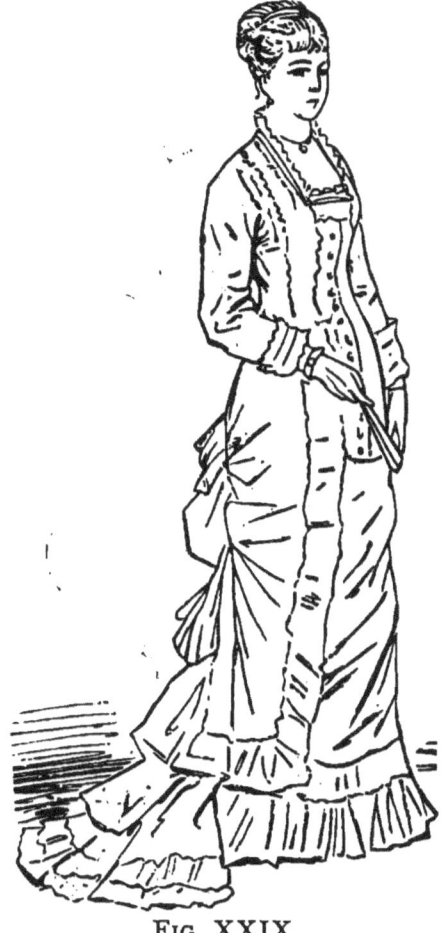

Fig. XXIX.

The most beautiful head, especially in woman, will be marred by an ungraceful carriage, as the finest foot, through a bad position, will lose the greater part of its beauty.

The shoulders must not be drawn upward or forward, but should be drawn somewhat backward, their horizontal line being preserved. On no account should we seek to emphasize tone

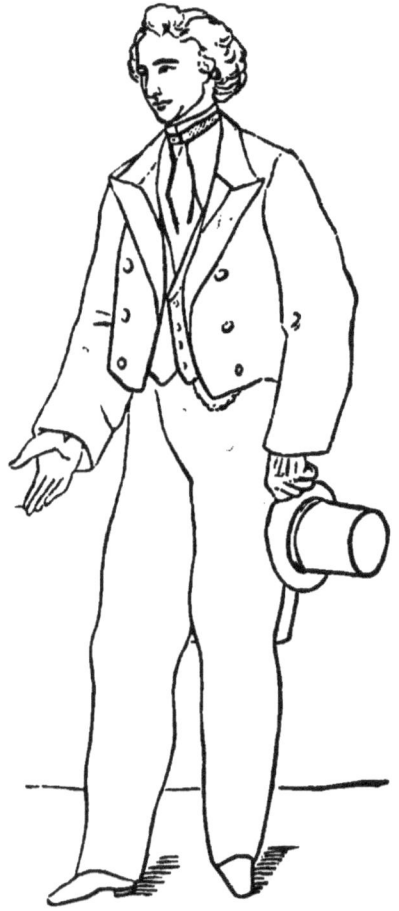

FIG. XXIX., *a*.

or word by a rising or falling of the shoulders. The shrug of the shoulders is, of course, excepted, as are also the few instances in which a movement of the shoulders is allowable. Among these are the representations of horror, or of sudden terror, in which the neck and head sink down between the raised shoulders.

Avoid a forced expansion of the chest, as it produces an impression of stiffness; still less must the chest be drawn inward. If this rule is strictly followed, crookedness of the back is impossible.

The abdomen should be drawn in somewhat. The arms must hang lightly and gracefully, and the drawing back of the elbows (a frequent fault in women) should be avoided. The carriage of the hands should be easy and unrestrained, the upper palms forward and the thumbs turned toward the thigh, yet in such a way that the thumb is visible (Fig. X.). In women the hands should be rather more forward (Fig. X., *d*).

In the "rococo age" the ladies held the hands in the following way: The upper arm was kept vertical, the lower arm hung lightly forward along the waist, and the right hand was laid on the left with its finger clasping it. This carriage of the hands is still, in our day, the most becoming. It is against the rules of decorum with both sexes to thrust the hands on the hips, or hold them crossed over the stomach, or lay them — in conversation with a person of higher rank — behind the back, or to thrust them into the pockets.

In the last century it was no breach of etiquette to place the hands inside the waistcoat; but they were never thrust into the pockets, least of all into the pockets of the pantaloons.

The fingers must be neither spread apart nor compressed, but each finger must keep its own place somewhat apart from the others; they should be bent but slightly, the index finger least, the little finger most of all.

The knees must not bend outward; neither must they be much drawn inward. In the one case laxness is indicated; in the other, stiffness.

When one addresses a person of his own rank, the feet generally assume the fourth position; when a person to whom he would pay deference, the first position. In the "rococo age" the feet were likewise held in the fourth position, but were brought nearer and nearer to the third, as the person addressed demanded more respect, until before a prince the third position was fully assumed, but never the first. (See Figs. LXVI. and LXVII.) This position was reserved only for soldiers and servants, or for persons receiving an order or a command.

3. Movement of the Arms and Hands.

Here all angularity and all parallels must be strictly avoided. Practice of the hand and arm exercises already given will ensure the student against these faults. Emphasizing what has been said on this subject, we proceed to treat of movements of the arms and hands. All such movements are based upon the *port de bras* of the art of dancing.

In every movement of the arms outward from the base position, the impulse to the movement, as we have already learned, should be given by the upper arm, which must appear to draw

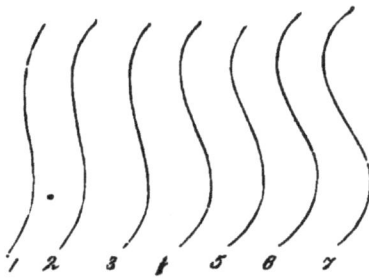

FIG. XXX.

the lower arm and hand after it. Any movement of the arms, to be truly plastic, must conform to Hogarth's line of beauty. Let us explain this line.

Of all lines, the wavy line has the purest æsthetic form; the

THE PLASTIC. 63

slight curvature, the gentle transition from one direction to another, make this line the most pleasing of all to the eye, and give it the first place in æsthetics. The wavy line can be varied infinitely. Hogarth, from a row of curved lines, the first of which curves but slightly, the next curving more, and so on, selects the middle line as the most perfect, and calls it *the line of beauty* (Fig. XXX., 4). Numbers 5, 6 and 7 become ungraceful because they curve too much, while numbers 3, 2 and 1 are too straight; hence 4 is the chosen line. Hogarth himself says of this wavy line: "It is known that bodies in motion always describe a line in the air. For example, the firebrand flung hastily creates a circle for every eye; the waterfall a curve; the ship upon the billows a wavy line, etc. So, also, the organic body when it moves entire, or only one limb. For instance, in break-

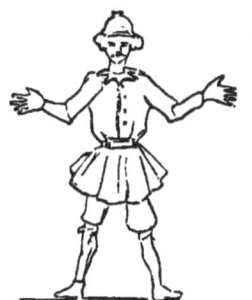

FIG. XXXI.

ing a wild, beautiful horse, which rushes on without a rider, we remark a long curve line in the way in which it sweeps through the air. This will all the more forcibly strike the eye in the human body, if we compare its movements with the straight lines of the puppet (Fig. XXXI.). The effect of the curve line may be noticed when one reaches a fan or some such object to a lady."

Figure XXXII. exhibits on the right hand side the angular puppet movements, as Figure XXXI., and on the left hand side the movements conforming to Hogarth's wavy line.

All movements of the arms, to be performed æsthetically, must conform to this line of beauty. Suppose, for example, that the hand (Fig. XXXII.) is to be moved from the base position to

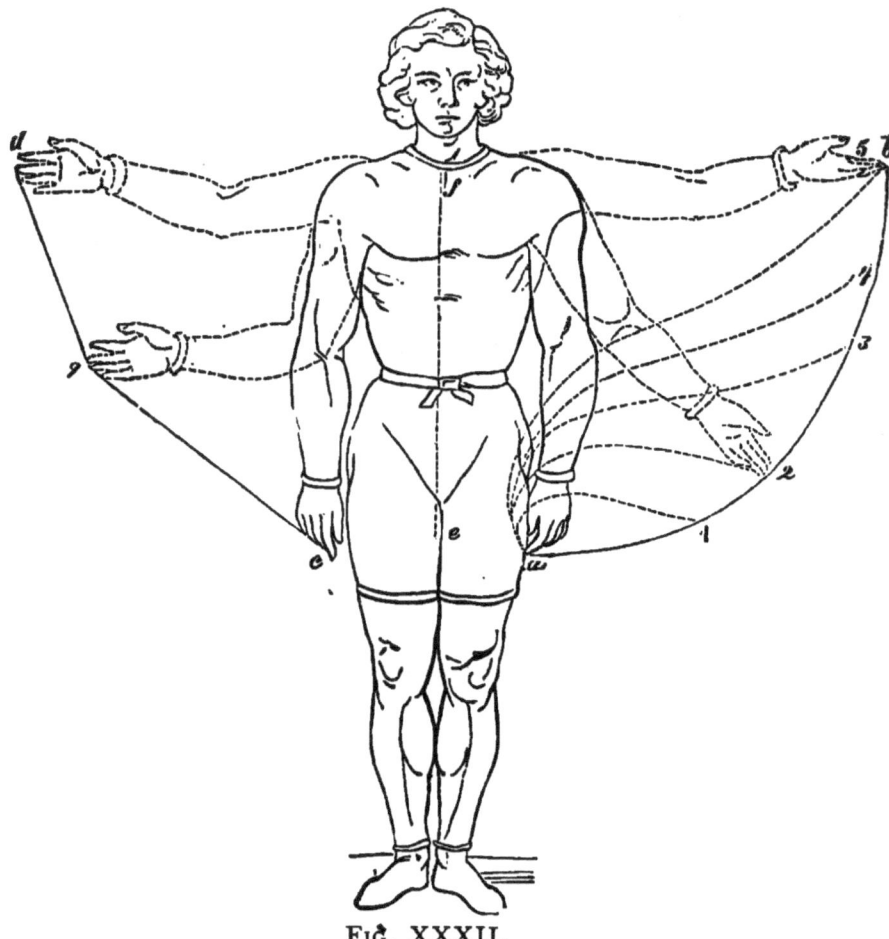

FIG. XXXII.

any of the five points marked down on the curved line *a–b;* the path of the movement must be none other than the dotted wavy line drawn to that point. If the hand is made to describe the straight lines *c–g*, *g–d*, we shall fall into the puppet movement (Fig. XXXI.). Even a repellent movement, whether great or slight, quick or slow, must take the direction of the wavy line.

This is the fundamental rule for all arm movements, and its various modifications arise only from the greater or less curvature of this line described by the hand. Beginners, and even those who have belonged for years to the stage, constantly offend the eye by following the straight lines *c*, *g*, *d*, in arm movements. Every one feels and derides the helplessness, angularity and absurd stiffness of this kind of movement without understanding its cause. If one understands the Hogarth line of beauty, he has reached a standpoint the attainment of which would require years without this knowledge. If he directs his movements in accordance with it, angularity and stiffness at once vanish.

When the arm falls back to its base position, the Hogarth line of beauty must also be strictly observed. While in every movement of the arm from the base position the impulse is given by the upper arm, in every movement back to the base position the hand must appear as giving the impulse.

The only way to the attainment of graceful, dignified movements, lies in the observance of these forms and their modifications, arising from situation, individuality, etc.

These lines need not be followed with school-boy conscientiousness and over-scrupulousness, but their main characteristics must be retained under all circumstances. Care must be taken not to make the wavy line too much curved or serpentine, as in Figure XXX., 7 ; and on the other hand one must avoid too slight curvature, which may degenerate into straight lines.

Let those who are inclined to deride all this as pedantry, observe the grace of a *danseuse*, her admirable ease and lightness, the round movements of her limbs, and reflect that without fundamental rules she could not have learned all this which so charms and delights us. She has so long practiced this one rule of Hogarth's that every movement has become facile and pleasing.

At the beginning of this book we declared utterly false that method of most teachers, who give certain studied movements for all human passions, whether joy or sorrow. All that is necessary is a *fundamental rule*, however pedantic it may appear to the superficial student. The finer shades must be sought out by him ; only in this way can he prove his originality.

Only when I know a theme perfectly, can I make variations upon it.

In plastic æsthetics it is not allowable, if simple, passionless emotions are to be depicted, to let the arm movement extend beyond the height of the shoulder. All emotions, which are not manifested in exalted language, must have their expression, so far as arm movements are concerned, inside of the following positions of the arm : The first, second and third *a* (see Fig.

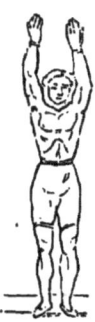

FIG. XXXIII.

LXVIII., *a*, the space between *a*, *d*, *e*, and Fig. XXVII., the space between 1 and 4), that is, within the limits the hands can describe from the base position, sideward and forward.

How ugly and unskilful is it when Tamino, in replying to the question, "Who will give us an answer?" accompanies the words

"The gods!" with the movement exhibited in Figure XXXIII., instead of making the movement in Figure XXXIV!

Passionate, eccentric emotions find their expression in the domain of the high *port de bras;* viz., in the third position (*b*) of the arms; that is, the arms, in such moments, pass beyond the shoulders over the space between *d, a, b* (Fig. LXVIII., *a*), and over the space 3 and 4 in Figure XXVII. These distinctions must be closely observed in dramatic representation, if one would work æsthetically.

The higher the position of the person, the lower and the less frequent will be the movements of the lower arms and hands; the lower the position, the more uncultured the person, the higher

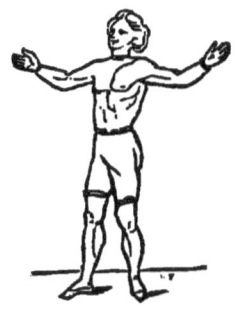

FIG. XXXIV.

and more frequent will be the movements. The man of culture, in general conversation, never allows the gesture to pass beyond the region of the shoulder.

The arm movements must not be jerky or inharmonious; they must proceed in gentle gradations one from the other. A piece of music should not be abruptly broken off; neither should an arm movement end suddenly. To use a musical simile, it should *die away,* except when horror or some sudden excitement ends it abruptly.

The nobler a person, the loftier his position, the more rounded and pleasing will be his movements; the more ignoble the person, the more unsymmetrical, angular and restless will they be. The first rule in arm movements is this: As little movement as possible. A French author says: "Dignity has no arms." These few words embody all rules.

If the hands are folded in front, one rule must be strictly observed: The folded arms must move only in the space described by the line *e–f*, Figure XXXII., and exceptionally in the third position *a* (see Fig. LXVIII., *a, a*).

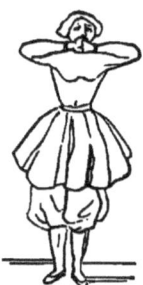

FIG. XXXV.

It is wholly false and contrary to all plastic rules to raise the clasped hands in front of the nose, with the elbows raised horizontally, as in Figure XXXV. Aside from the fact that this is unplastic, it hides the expression of the face, which is the main thing at such moments. The highest point to which the clasped hands may be carried, is *f* in Figure XXXII.

If the arms are extended imploringly, they must not pass beyond the point just designated. Care must be taken that the elbows do not protrude sideways, but remain as in Figure XXXVI. Only in moments of despair is it allowable to raise the clasped hands above the head. In this case, when they reach the level of the face, they are inverted, the palms upward without being separated, the fingers remaining clasped, and are thus lifted above the head.

To avoid parallels with the arms and hands (Fig. XXXVII.), care should be taken, while in action, to have one arm and hand in a different position from the other (Fig. XXXVIII.).

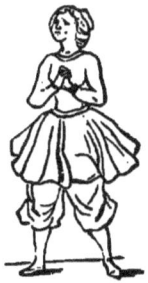

FIG. XXXVI.

When the hand is placed upon the breast, as in protestation, the fingers should be in their natural position, neither far apart nor pressed closely together. The hand should be placed upon

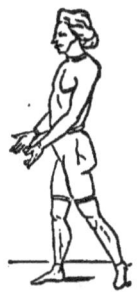

FIG. XXXVII.

the heart, and not, as constantly happens, upon the bosom. If both hands are laid upon the chest, one should be in the region of the heart, the other above it, as in Figure XXXIX., *a*.

We may be allowed to refer to many violations of this rule, as well as to some *gaucheries*, which are altogether too frequent.

Many young actors seem to be in doubt as to where their internal organs lie. When, for instance, Tamino sings, "I feel it," placing his right hand passionately upon the left shoulder, and extending the elbow horizontally, as in Figure XL., one would infer that his heart lies there. Or when Pamina sings, "Ah, I feel it! It has vanished!" and instead of simply placing one or both hands on her heart, covers her bosom with her hands, and

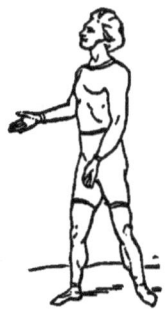

FIG. XXXVIII.

in that region where the neck begins (Fig. XLI.). What shall we say of Pamina's feelings?

There are so many of these faults that we need only mention them to warn our readers against them:

Constant rubbing of the hands.

Planting the hands in the sides.

Thrusting them into the pockets.

Biting the nails, or gazing at them to relieve an embarrassed pause.

Twirling the thumbs.

Plucking at the furniture or other objects around, or at people.

Toying with or pulling at the button of the person to whom one is speaking.

Trifling with one's watch chain.

Folding the hands across the back under the coat-tails, etc.

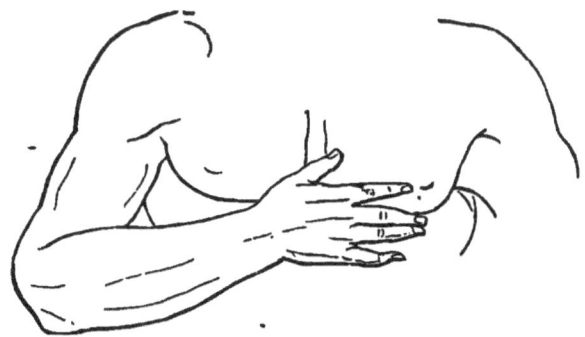

FIG. XXXIX.

Nothing but incessant practice of the *port de bras*, as given in Figure XXVII., will enable one to execute the arm movements easily and gracefully according to the rules laid down. When

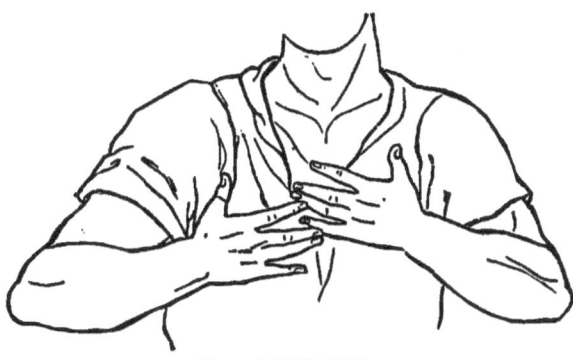

FIG. XXXIX., *a*.

this has been done so thoroughly that the whole comes to the pupil without effort, he may be certain that his movements will be neither stiff, angular, clumsy nor awkward, unless he makes them so designedly. At the slightest ungainly movement, he must recall the fundamental rule, which must have become so

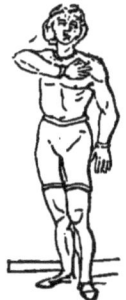

Fig. XL.

much a part of him that his movements will be involuntary — an outcome of his very life. No actor should appear before the public before becoming a perfect master of these arm movements.

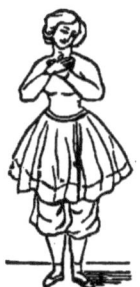

Fig. XLI.

The public, which pays its entrance fee, should not be tortured with bad gymnastic efforts dictated by no rule, and which, save in a few exceptional cases, can produce no true æsthetic movement.

THE PLASTIC.

MOVEMENTS.

1. *Walking in General.*

We know the mechanism of walking, and shall now consider it from an æsthetic standpoint. It is important to note that, in walking, the body is not thrown to and fro, or back and forth, at every step, but that the leg movements, beginning at the hips, in no way affect the upper part of the body which only inclines slightly forward. A certain equality must also be observed in the length of the steps and the *tempo;* that is, short and long steps must not alternate, as this makes the gait awkward or affected.

Among the faults to be avoided are:

Walking with stiff legs.

Walking with a too rapid uplifting of the toes or heels.

Walking with a decidedly forward inclination of the upper part of the body.

A tripping gait.

A dancing, skipping gait.

Walking as if upon india-rubber soles.

A stiff gait.

Walking with the arms held stiffly forward, or moved about too much.

Too rapid a gait.

A creeping, or slipping gait.

Too heavy a step, etc.

We need not dwell upon these bad habits; it suffices to name them.

2. *The Walking of Ladies with Trains.*

Who has not often seen in private life, as well as on the stage, ladies with long trains, who at every half-dozen steps seemed on the point of falling by stepping on their own clothes? We have witnessed this with the firm conviction that it could not be remedied, that the unfortunate ladies must yield to their fate. But a little consideration of our rules in regard to walking will explain the reason of all this. These ladies do not walk right; they set down the back of the heel first, and then the toes; their gait lacks energy. This stepping upon the dress may be easily avoided.

What an aspect would an Iphigenia present if, upon stepping forward in her sacred grove, while holding up her veil artistically with one hand, she should lift her robe in front with the other, or step upon it repeatedly, in beginning her monologue:

"Out here in your shadows, etc."

But how can such a defect be avoided? Simply by setting down the lower part of the heel and the ball of the foot at the same time, and making the forward step with decided energy, with the toes turned outward, and yet held firmly downward, as if the person would push her skirts before her at every step. If the heel is first set upon the floor, or if the required energy is wanting, treading upon the dress is unavoidable, and no trembling or wishing that this may not happen, will prevent it.

A lady versed in ordinary walking, should practice walking in trained robes, otherwise, whether she belong to the stage or to the *salon*, she will not produce the impression of *noblesse*.

The walk backward is executed in the manner already described in Part First, but care must be taken that the toes are turned outward as far as possible, and at every step the dress must be lifted with the side of the foot. The feet must be set back somewhat obliquely, and not in a direct line.

My lady pupils have found these rules of great practical benefit. Many who have long been connected with the stage, assure me, that anxiety lest they might step upon their dresses, has caused the failure of many a rôle.

This practice in long dresses must be followed until such ease is acquired, that it would seem as if the ladies had never worn any other. Most ladies now give the impression of appearing in a trained robe for the first time. Whether upon the stage or in the *salon*, a lady should seem to be perfectly at home and in her own sphere.

3. *The Lifting of a Lady's Dress in Walking.*

To lift the dress on both sides at once is awkward and unsightly. In lifting the skirt, it should be taken lightly between the thumb and forefinger, and gathered into graceful folds with the other fingers, the arm being drawn somewhat forward. This is the most pleasing and decorous way of lifting the dress. The train must be so held that the lining does not come outside, and the underskirts are not visible.

4. *Turning to the Right and Left in Walking.*

In changing one's direction in walking, one foot must not be set over the other, but the foot on the side to which one turns must take the first step in the new direction. The turning is performed on the ball of the stationary foot.

5. *Turning to the Right or Left while Standing.*

If in standing between two persons, one has to speak to each alternatively, he turns upon the balls of both feet, lifting only the heel from the floor, so that on the right hand side the right foot and on the left hand side the left foot, stands in the fourth position. All grace vanishes, if, in turning from right to left or *vice versa*, several steps are taken.

6. *Walking Sideward.*

If one has to take several side steps, he extends the foot sideway and without turning the body (second position), drawing the other foot into the fifth position or beyond it, behind the foot that is set sideway; he then passes again into the second position, drawing the other foot up into the first. It looks very awkward to turn the whole body for two side steps; as when they are made, it must naturally turn again. Ladies with long trains must carefully observe these precepts.

7. *Stepping Sideward with Bowing.*

If one has to make an obeisance while stepping to one side, he must take two steps while turning the body, and make the bow. The first step is not taken in the second position, but in the fourth, the centre of gravity being carried over to this foot, while the other foot passes into the fifth position behind the first, which is thereupon placed in the second position to prepare the bow. If the movement demands more than the two steps, then in this case, also, the foot first moved is placed in the fourth position, but the other foot, instead of being carried back into the fifth position, is only brought into the first and, without being set down, makes a backward step, followed by others as the occasion requires. The last step (the one preparatory to bowing), is taken sideward in the second position; the other foot then passes into the first position, and the bow is made.

With our modern ladies, the last step is not a sideward step, but the foot which is drawn back last is placed in the third position, and the bow immediately follows; *i. e.*, the knees are bent, one foot drawn back and the other drawn after it. (See the modern compliment, Part Fourth.)

8. *Turning Round in Walking.*

If one has to turn round in walking, the turning should be done on the balls of the feet toward the side of the posterior foot, the heels being slightly elevated. It is entirely wrong, in turning, to set the foremost foot over the other, and it is contrary to every æsthetic law.

If the actor strides across the whole breadth of the stage, and has to turn and retrace his steps, he must turn with his face to the audience; that is, the foot nearest the audience must, at the moment, be the posterior one. To turn, as it were, on his own axis, and with his back to the audience, is allowable only when the situation demands it.

Although the barriers have fallen which, half a century ago,

THE PLASTIC.

forbade the dramatic actor to turn his back to the public, and a more free and natural movement is now allowable, the laws of beauty have not vanished from the stage — must never vanish from it. Many things may be permitted, but still be ungainly. We shall refer to this subject again.

9. *Turning Round while Standing.*

Turning round while standing must be performed this way: If the person stands in the fourth position, he should always turn toward the side of the hindmost foot. While the foremost foot turns upon the ball, the other foot remains upon the ball during only half the revolution, the other half being made on the heel, the toes being turned outward. If one stands with the heels in contact (first position) before turning, one foot must take a slight step backward, and the turning ensue toward this side the same instant.

10. *Turning in the Case of Women.*

If a lady wears a dress with a train, the following rules must be strictly observed: If she stands in the fourth position with the right foot forward, before turning, this foot must be brought into the fourth position backward, and with such force that the train is thrust backward somewhat, and out of the way. The turning then takes place upon the ball of the foot just set back, the other foot resting upon the heel. The right foot must not now take the first step, since, in this case, she would be sure to step upon her train; but the left foot must take its first step in a half-sideway, half-forward direction.

If the lady stands in the fourth position with the left foot forward, this foot must pass backward and the turning take place toward the left. If she stands in the first, second, or third position, the step which one of the two feet takes backward must be longer than usual, and more decided. The stepping forward, after turning, takes place in the same way as already described.

A pulling of the train to the right or left in lifting it, indicates that one is unaccustomed to the wearing of such a dress. Those ladies only who avoid this and similar faults, and move gracefully in such clothes, will make us believe that they are accustomed to wear them.

11. *Carriage of the Arms in Walking.*

We constantly notice an awkwardness in the carriage of the arms while walking, especially in young girls. It is that stiff, falling of the arms forward, and their machine-like jerking up and down at every step. The arms belong to the side of the body; and, if ladies are allowed to carry their arms somewhat farther forward, this is only when in repose (Fig. X., *a*). In walking, the arms, unless they have something to do, must swing lightly and gracefully at the side.

12. *The Opening of a Door.*

If one has to open a door from the outside, if the knob is at his left, he should grasp it with the right hand, holding his hat in his left; the right foot should stand upon the threshold, the left being somewhat in the rear, and sustaining the centre of gravity. As he opens the door, the right foot takes the first short step into the room, the left foot the second. As the centre of gravity has now fallen back upon the left foot, and the right foot has resumed the first position, the right hand, which has, until now, held the door-knob, should let go of it, leaving the door behind. He now steps to the left into the second sideway-forward position, and using this step as a preparation for compliments, the bow follows with a drawing forward of the right foot.

By taking a third step into the room, one passes beyond the reach of the door and avoids that constantly recurring fatality of having it thrust against one's back by the person entering immediately after.

If, on entering, the door-knob is on the right, all these movements should, of course, be reversed.

If one, in departing, has to open a door from within, he should step back to the door into the position in which he stood after taking the second step upon his entrance. Now, bowing his adieu, he should grasp the door-knob from behind with the hand next to it, and step backward over the threshold, in the same manner as upon his entrance, letting go the inner knob, and closing the door with the outer one.

Women should enter in the same manner, only that one more step is required.

Great care must be taken to learn these rules. A person is characterized by his mere silent entrance into a room.

13. The Entrance of a Servant.

If a servant enters the presence of his master or mistress, he never pays any compliments; when he withdraws, he does so without bowing. (This rule is constantly violated upon the stage.) The servant allows every one he ushers in to precede him, and then follows. When he announces a visitor, and receives permission for him to enter, he does not open the door from within; he leaves the room and opens it from without. If a servant enters a strange room, as soon as the door closes he takes a step to one side in the second position, passing beyond range of the door, and remaining there until he has done his errand, excepting when he has something to deliver; in which case he advances to within one step's distance of the person to whom he is sent.

14. The Setting of a Chair for One's Self or for Others.

If one has to set a chair, he does not take it by one side, but, stepping behind it, grasps the back with both hands, so that the thumbs shall come forward, the index fingers upon the side, and the three other fingers behind its back. He then lifts it from the floor, and passes to the appointed place (Fig. XLII.).

If a servant has to set a chair, he sets it down lightly and then steps back. If one sets a chair for himself, he takes it to within two steps of the required place. (The rank of the person near whom he sets it, determines the distance.) He then sets the chair down lightly, first upon the fore feet, then with his eyes

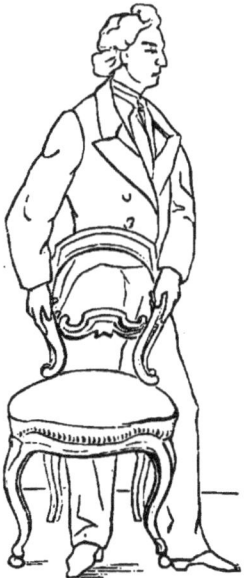

FIG. XLII.

fixed upon the person near whom he is about to sit, he steps in in front of the chair and sits down (Fig. XLIII.).

15. Seating One's Self upon a Chair already Placed.

The general rule is as follows; its finer shades must be left to each individual:

For Gentlemen.— If the chair is at the left, as in Figure XLIII., one places himself beside it in the first position; then takes a step forward with the right foot, carrying the other foot into the first and without stepping into the second position, to the front of the chair. Then, with his face toward the person near whom he is to seat himself, he lets himself easily down upon the middle of the chair, without leaning against its back.

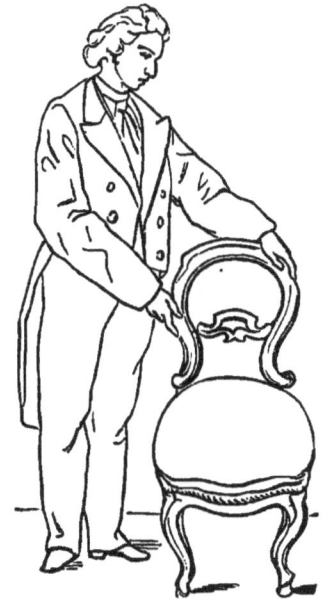

FIG. XLIII.

In sitting between two persons, one of whom is of higher rank than the other, the face should be turned more toward the first; if between a gentleman and a lady, the lady has the preference.

To look around at the chair, before sitting down, is highly improper.

The sitting down must not be hasty. The body must be as erect as possible, without stiffness.

If one has a sword at his side, in sitting down he draws it forward with the left hand; when seated, he lets it glide back to his side.

It is not allowable to draw the coat-tails forward with both hands before sitting down, unless in the slightest degree, and without occasioning remark. It is better left undone, as is the practice with all polished gentlemen.

For Ladies.— Ladies who, in the costume of the "rococo" age, cannot feel the chair on account of their hooped skirts, find it very difficult to seat themselves well. There is constant danger of shoving the chair back with their skirts. They must, therefore, exactly measure the distance before sitting down, and take their backward steps accordingly. Before seating themselves they should draw the dress slightly forward with the hand farthest from the person near whom they are to be seated, letting it fall again at the side. The other hand should be held in readiness for the possibility of the chair being shoved backward. In this case they must grasp the back of the chair from behind. If a lady seats herself upon a sofa, or anything firm, she can use both hands in drawing her skirts forward slightly from the sides, letting them fall back as soon as she is seated.

It is decidedly "bad form" to draw the skirts forward with each hand alternately, prior to sitting down. It is just as inadmissible in rising to grasp them from behind, and to seek, through all sorts of movements, to restore them to order. If a lady has seated herself in the way prescribed, upon rising she can let her dress fall quietly back into its natural position without fear of its disarrangement.

16. Kneeling.

In order to kneel and rise properly one should often practice the exercises given for *strengthening the muscles.* (Part Second.)

Kneeling takes place in this way : One steps, as circumstances require, more or less near the person before whom he is to kneel, bending the knee of one leg while he allows the other to glide back slowly or quickly, with the foot turned outward, the great toe only passing over the floor. The line of gravity falls upon the foremost leg, only a slight fraction coming upon the toes of the other leg, which is shoved backward. Then one sinks upon the knee of the backward leg, which (upon the stage) should be turned toward the audience. The lower part of the forward leg should neither form an acute angle with the upper which happens if the knee is pressed too far forward; nor an obtuse angle, which happens if the foot is set too far forward; it should form a right angle. The foot of the kneeling leg should not have its toes turned downward and inward, but outward and backward as in Figure LXXVIII. The upper part of the body should be held as erect as possible, but not stiff.

Rising should take place with the aid of both legs, which should elevate the body in such a way that the line of gravity may fall in the middle of the base described by the two feet.

If the body is so far erect that the foremost foot may sustain the centre of gravity alone, the hindmost foot is drawn slowly forward; but not *vice versa*.

If one rises quickly with the upper body bent forward, the person standing in front will almost inevitably be inconvenienced.

If one has to kneel before an exalted personage, from whom he has received some favor, or whose hand he wishes to kiss, he should at first approach within the distance of one step, and then fall on his knees in the manner indicated.

To kneel two or three steps away from the person, is awkward and contrary to etiquette.

Kneeling on both legs is allowable in the following cases:

(*a*) In the prayers of Roman Catholics, where this is required.
(*b*) In moments of exalted passion.
(*c*) In extreme old age.
(*d*) By slaves, as to denote the utmost degree of humiliation.
(*e*) In country people.
(*f*) In representing comic situations, mostly by servants and chambermaids.

If one would rise, from his kneeling posture (on both knees), the foot turned from the public first assumes the position it had when kneeling upon one knee, in which case the rising in a decorous way comes as a matter of course; while, in opposite cases, the effect is unpleasant.

In falling upon both knees, the upper part of the body should not bend forward, as one might easily fall over, but it should, as far as possible, sink directly into the knee.

17. Lifting Something from the Floor.

If something is to be lifted from the floor or laid down, this should not happen in a sort of cowering posture, with the upper body bent forward and downward (unless this is demanded in personation), but as in kneeling by bending the leg turned away from the public, and by shoving back the other leg which is toward the public, and upon the knee of which one falls.

The rising takes place as directed under the head of "Kneeling."

In a rapid execution of the aforesaid movement, the leg that is shoved backward does not come at all into a full kneeling posture; but while it is shoved back, the forward leg bends inward quickly, almost wholly bearing the weight of the body; and again stretches itself with the elasticity of a spring, while the backward leg is just as quickly drawn forward.

The knee-exercises given in "Physical Gymnastics," now come into play, it being almost impossible to execute the movements here given without this practice.

18. Falling upon the Stage.

The finer shades of such falling are as various as the motives inciting the actor to fall. An attempt to describe them would be absurd, but a fundamental rule derived from long experience as an actor, will be in place here.

Let the motive for falling be what it may, the actor should always begin to fall from the feet, in accordance with the fundamental rule, that is, he should always first set the muscles that rule the foot and knee-joints out of action, thus sinking into his knees (which for the most part happens sideward), and then let the upper part of the body fall. In falling forward or backward, this main rule must also be observed. In falling forward, it must be noted that both arms, stretched forward, reach the floor sooner than the face, serving as a sort of protection; in falling sideward, it will be one arm.

19. *The Holding of the Hat.*

In our time which is distinguished by freedom of manners and indifference to the rules of etiquette, there are no fixed rules as to how the gentleman who remains for a long time uncovered, must hold or carry his hat. But in any event, the following may be stated as a rule: Let a gentleman hold his hat as he will, he always exactly observes *one* rule: *he does not shift it from one hand to the other;* this betrays the man without *tournure* in private life, and upon the stage the uncultured artist. The simplest and most decorous way of holding the hat is this: One takes with the thumb, the index and middle fingers, that part of the brim which covers the forehead, and in this manner carries the hat to one side, so that the inner surface is turned toward the thigh, the arm hanging in its natural position at the side (Fig. XXIX., a). It is awkward to hold the hat before one so that those standing opposite can see into it. Neither should the hat be taken by the inside, as the cleanest hat is liable to soil the gloves or hands.

In saluting a person you meet, for instance on the right, take the hat from the head with the left hand, and *vice versa*. While you stand before this person with uncovered head, the hand holding the hat should hang at the side, its inner rim turned toward the dress.

Actors should bear in mind that in the "rococo" time (age of Louis XIV., XV., and XVI. in France) if one took the hat into the *salon*, he carried it under the left arm in the manner above described, but never with the hand hanging down at the side. If he had a *chapeau claque*, he also held it with part of the brim hanging downward before him, and with part of it between the thumb and finger of each hand. Servants only carried the hat in the one hand hanging at the side.

20. *The Carrying of the Fan.*

The use of the fan is very ancient, and comes from Asia and Africa, where palm-leaves were used at first, and peacock and other feathers at a later day. Its purpose was to protect the face from the sun or to move the air.

In the Orient, the larger fans are borne by slaves before or near those who use them; each person holding a small fan himself. A Chinese host, when the heat is great, after the tea has been drunk, takes a fan and holding it in both hands, says: "I invite you to use the fan." Each guest then takes his fan. It would be impolite for the host to have none, for then no guest would use his fan. In Greece and Rome the host made the air cool by using the fan himself or having his slaves use it. Very costly fans were carried in the middle ages. Their use was so general, that the fan became an indispensable necessity to every well-bred young lady. A genuine fan-language arose and reached its height in the last century. The French Revolution abolished the fan, and only in recent times has it become the necessary adjunct of the fine lady.

Although the artistic handling of the fan, which characterized ladies of the past century, is not demanded of those of the present day, still we may at least demand that the lady who carries a fan, shall not swing it around uselessly in the air, or use it in an awkward manner.

As in gesture, repose is always made the main principle; this applies also to the use of the fan. It is to be used either for moving the air, or to be held quietly in the hand as a mere ornament. But the manner of holding it must always indicate ease and a knowledge of polite usage, else one does better not to carry it at all.

We find in Mereau's little work the simplest and most decorous manner of carrying the fan: "The fan must be so held between the thumb and index finger of the right hand, that its upper edge falls downward. Some ladies hold their fans straight before them, and in such a way that the upper edge almost touches the chin. Others hold the fan under the left arm, or horizontally before them. These various methods are all alike faulty and in direct contradiction to that genuine fine breeding we expect in a lady of culture."

If a lady lets the upper right arm fall perpendicularly to the hip, the lower arm being somewhat bent, the position of the fan-holding arm will be the true one for an attitude of repose (Fig. XXIX.). Every movement of the fan out of this attitude should be made with the wrist, and not by the aid of the whole lower arm (much less of the upper arm). Even if the movement becomes greater, and the whole arm takes part in it, the main stress must lie in the wrist.

Here the necessity of wrist practice, as given in Part Second, becomes evident. Without it every movement of the fan will be a forced movement.

21. *Carrying a Cane.*

If one carries a cane on account of lameness or general weakness, no directions are needed. He will carry it as the nature of the malady demands. If fashion or one's own pleasure is the motive, it is quite otherwise. In such a case one should avoid shifting the cane from one hand to the other, placing it across the back or over the shoulders, flourishing it in the air, etc. If it is a light walking cane, and is carried for pleasure, a playful movement is admissible; but with a stout cane all useless movement should be avoided, and the carrying of the cane given an impression of the utmost ease.

The actor, in carrying a cane, should be still more circumspect. Above all, he should avoid carrying it outside the theatre. Even Goethe lays down this law. All too easily does he become accustomed to it, and its lack will cause him great annoyance on the stage. If neglected, the actor will contract bad habits which will annoy him upon the stage. How often do we see the actor with the hand that usually carries the cane, restless and ill at ease, seeking to make movements, until he remembers that he is upon the stage.

The actor should form no habits which he cannot renounce upon the stage. Carrying a cane is allowed him only when the character or situation demands or allows it. But he should always proceed from the fundamental rule that the bearing of the cane is to have its significance to the spectators. He must use all outward appliances sparingly, such as canes, eye-glasses, etc.; otherwise he weakens their significance. In their use he should discriminate exactly whether he represents a personality which actually requires them, or one which only coquets with them. In the former case, he brings the glass directly before his eye without marked preparation; in the latter with more or less marked movement and affectation.

In the seventeenth and eighteenth centuries the cane was an adjunct of full dress, and played a distinguished *rôle*. It was a huge Spanish reed with a gold head and tassel; was grasped under the head and borne usually in a dignified manner.

22. *The Use of the Handkerchief.*

While, in every-day life, one only takes his handkerchief in his hand when he really needs it, we see that upon the stage this often happens unnecessarily. With ladies this is excusable, partly because it is a usual custom to carry the handkerchief in the hand, and partly because the handkerchief (often embroidered with lace) is considered a requisite of the toilet. But what shall we say of a gentleman who is always seen upon the stage with handkerchief in hand, passing it from one hand to the other, from breast-pocket to coat and other pockets, taking it out the next moment, to pass it over mouth or beard — one who even gesticulates in presence of ladies with handkerchief in hand? This indecorum has so passed into a habit with many actors that they cannot play certain *rôles* without the handkerchief.

It is only a fop or a fool, young or old, who takes out his handkerchief every moment to use it as just described. The actor of fine culture does this only when the author's purpose demands it (for unforeseen surprises, to represent bleeding at the nose, to dry the forehead, etc.); but never to trifle with it, and that in the presence of ladies.

Neither is it allowable for the actor to take out the handkerchief to dry his tears. In the first place, a man does not weep; in the second place, if the stage business actually demands that a few tears be shed, he does not dry them with a handkerchief. Here propriety allows women what it denies to men.

The gradations of the real purpose which renders a handkerchief necessary, are allowed only to the comic actor or soubrette, and that only in rare cases.

23. *The Hand-kiss,*

as a token of respect or reverence, demands several degrees in its execution, which must be determined by the rank of the person who kisses, as well as by that of the one whose hand is kissed. This is a specialty in acting. We consider the hand-kiss from the æsthetic-plastic standpoint, and hereby present it in two forms:

(*a*) *The Hand-kiss of Thanks, of Entreaty for Forgiveness, of Gallantry, of Lovers.*— Here the one who kisses, takes the hand of the person kissed, lifts it slightly from the normal position, bows down to it, and presses the kiss inaudibly upon it. It is exceedingly ill-bred to draw the hand forward without bending down to it, and then press the kiss upon it; or to let the kiss be audible. This always indicates the man devoid of fine tact. If the lady's hand is covered with a glove, the hand is not kissed, but the wrist. In case the lady stands at the right, the right hand of the gentleman grasps her left hand; if she stands at the left, his left grasps her right hand. In this sort of a kiss the normal position is usually retained, and yet with a slight variation if love, reverence or gratitude dictate the kiss. The lover, in his passion, will raise the hand of the beloved somewhat higher, and only bend slightly himself, while, in the first case, the hand is raised only a little, and a full inclination toward it takes place.

(*b*) In the hand-kiss of etiquette, especially that of a lower person to a higher, up to a crowned head, the one who kisses should in no case grasp the hand and raise it. It will be held out to him, and he slips his hand (the index finger uppermost) under the hand he is to kiss so that his own forms support, and, without drawing the proffered hand out of its position in the slightest degree, he imprints the kiss upon it. Slight gradations enter here, as everywhere, on account of higher or lower rank. To designate these would be absurd, even impossible. We have only given the fundamental rules.

24. Fundamental Rules for Position if Several Persons are on the Stage.

If several persons on the stage engage in conversation, the æsthetic plastic demands that this happen in accordance with one rule, which is simply as follows: If two persons standing near each other have to converse a long time, they must take especial care to avoid the profile attitude, through which the sound of their words in the *coulisses* is wholly lost. The speaker should stand somewhat back of the listener, so that at least three-fourths of his face and figure are toward the audience; while the listener, without incurring the reproach of stiffness or unnaturalness, may stand opposite the public — if only the intention of listening is expressed by head and gesture. Both actors would do well to follow the above rule, so that the speaker, as soon as he ends, may lightly and unremarked, take half a step before the listener, who recedes half a step. Naturally, this can happen only in more weighty discourse; in brief, disjointed conversation, both stand with three-fourths profile to the public, without stepping forward or backward. It is exceedingly unpleasant to have both actors, when standing near each other, turn their faces directly to the audience reminding one of puppets which can move only upon one line. Such situations may happen, yet they should be but momentary.

If three or more persons stand near one another, this must never be in a direct line (drawn from one side of the stage to the other), but always in a semi-circle. (Figs. XLIV. and XLV.) If

FIG. LXIV.   FIG. LXV.

six, eight or more persons are upon the stage, and all take part in one conversation, they may, to avoid the monotony of one large semi-circle, form single groups of three or four in small half-circles; but all these must lie within the periphery of the large half-circle. (Fig. XLVI.)

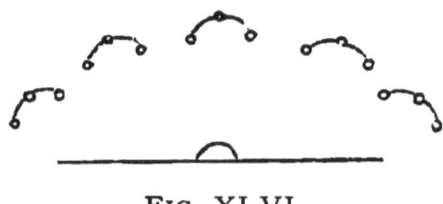

FIG. XLVI.

This figure shows fifteen persons, forming five single groups; and yet the whole fifteen, in this position, represent but one group. What an aspect would they present to the æsthetic eye, did they stand in a straight line, as in Figure XLVII., or in one

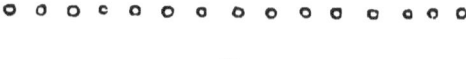

FIG. XLVII.

convex to the public, as in the lines which appear in Figure XLVIII! Would they not give an impression of the utmost awkwardness and stiffness? The semi-circle, on the other hand, is always agreeable to the æsthetic eye.

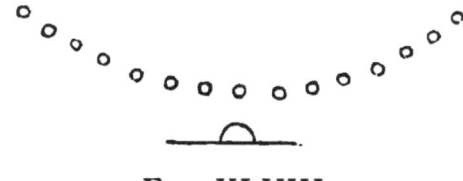

FIG. XLVIII.

25. *Position of Subordinates.*

The German manner of having subordinates always stand in the rear (thus obliging the higher personages to turn around), has already been deprecated by Ludwig Schröder in his "Precepts of the Actor's Art."

Let this hero of the German stage speak for himself: "If a servant announces some one, he certainly remains at the door, receives his orders and makes his exit. This is grounded in our customs. But for him who is allowed entrance, whoever he may be, there is upon the stage no front or rear, or in other words, he is subordinate to him who stands nearer the footlights. By this position he facilitates the speech and play of the leading character."

CHAPTER II.

THE MIMIC ART.

> "All our movements are merely automatic, and express nothing if the face meantime remains dumb, and does not lend them soul and life."—
> NOVERRE'S LETTERS.

INTRODUCTION.

Mimic art is either the talent for imitating certain individuals by modifications of one's own body, or the art of conforming outward appearances to ideas which represent inward emotions. It is divided (1) into face-movements — play of the features, and (2) into movements of the whole body or certain parts of it — the play of gesture.

True to the purpose of this book, we give only main principles. Those who would gain a thorough knowledge of these subjects, may study Engel's excellent work, "Ideas upon Acting;" Dr. Piderit's "Principles of Mimic Art and Physiognomy," and Seckendorf's "Lectures on Mimic Art and Declamation."

PLAY OF FEATURES.

1. General Remarks.

The human organism has the capability of appropriating outward impressions, and expressing their effect in the lineaments of the face. Men are distinguished from one another by the greater or less measure of this capability. Hence the features of the face are the hand-writing of the soul. The more lively a man's fancy and the more cultured his mind, the easier will be to him the reception of outward impressions, and the mirroring them in the features of the face. The actor, who does not actually receive the impulse for the expression to be reproduced, from the outside, must possess the liveliest imagination in order to reproduce its effect in his facial lineaments. Hence it necessarily follows that those only can be actors who possess this peculiarity in a high degree. To seek to acquire it by the aid of fixed rules is a vain attempt.

A lively fancy allows all impressions, voluntary and involuntary, to enter into the features ; when such a fancy is lacking, all description of the muscles of the face and their manner of working is useless, and must result only in most complete caricature.

This play of features is produced by the muscles of the face; hence a round, full face with its muscles all enveloped in fat, is little calculated to mirror the emotions of the soul. Only the eyes are left it, and important as these are in expression they will not suffice alone.

The actor's first task is to acquire ability to keep the facial muscles in perfect repose. Every sitting for a photographer, teaches us how difficult this is. The proper method is to practice before a mirror, first single muscles, seeking perfect repose for each, or to move each group of muscles singly (as those of the mouth), taking care that no grimace appears. When a sufficient degree of mobility has been brought into the muscles of the face, one endeavors to express all passions in his mien, having first gained a perfect mental grasp of each. If he would express sorrow, joy, etc., he holds the features fixed for a moment before gazing into the mirror, to see whether the muscles of the face obey, or whether they must be aided in some way. The features must always be noble, not losing this character even in the highest passion. Eyes and mouth are most important in this play of the features.

2. *The Eyes.*

"The eye is the mirror of the soul." The eye shows us the manner in which the impression on the soul is gradually developed. Its importance is self-evident. The man with a cold, staring or indifferent eye, had best renounce the idea of going upon the stage ; it will not be possible for him to awaken sympathy or convince his audience that he feels the truth of what he says.

If an actor wears spectacles, and takes them off, his eyes will wander around without expression; it will be difficult, almost impossible, for him to give them expression. If one has naturally wide-open eyes he must be circumspect in the portrayal of simple emotions lest an unpleasant sharpness or a rigid stare enter his glance, when he opens his eyes still wider. The manner of entirely closing the eyes, of uttering whole sentences, now and then suddenly opening the eyes, is quite unpardonable. There is a play of the features where a lowering of the lids so that the eyes seem closed, is effective ; but this must not become stereotyped. In this case the spectator does not see several individuals personified ; he sees only the individuality of the actor. Too great mobility of the eyebrows must also be guarded against, and likewise that constant contraction of the forehead which may easily become a grimace.. It is not allowable to let the eyes sweep around the audience, or rest here and there upon the boxes. In this way all semblance of truth is lost.

3. The Mouth.

Next to the eyes, the mouth has the greatest significance in the play of the features. When all the muscles of the mouth are in normal tension, the mouth line is waving and beautiful. (Fig. XLIX.) In this position all undue tension of the muscles is to be avoided; in speaking and singing this must also be guarded against,. else the mouth may assume a forced or even ignoble expression. Many actors have the mistaken idea that in speaking, the mouth must make motions similar to those of the tongue. As a result of this, we see carp-like movements of the lips become chronic, while their sole task should be to form the labials by mere opening and closing, the vowels (*o* and *oo*) by a slight rounding.

In the portrayal of scorn, malignity, contempt, weeping, etc., in which the corners of the mouth especially are active, care must be taken not to draw down the mouth too much or have the tension too great. In conclusion, we must warn against one constantly recurring fault, viz.: Opening the mouth involuntarily in effective situations, and letting it remain open. This might be allowable only in comic acting.

In the portrayal of difficulty of hearing or of listening, it is proper to open the mouth, for in both instances the reverberation is sought not only through the ear but also through the mouth, which, by means of the eustachian tube, stands in connection with the auditory passage.

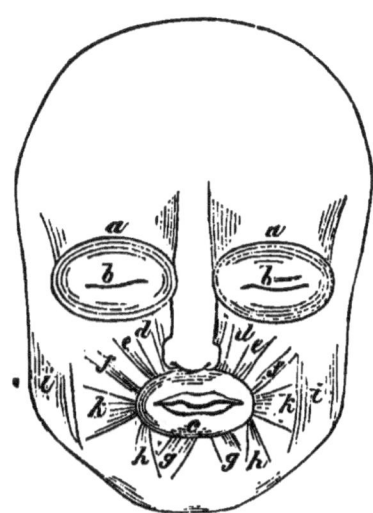

FIG. XLIX.

MUSCLES OF THE FACE.

a, a, occipito-frontalis; *b, b*, orbicularis palpebrarum; *c*, orbicularis oris; *d, d*, levator labii superioris alæque nasi; *e, e*, levator labii superioris proprius; *f, f*, zygomaticus major; *k, k*, buccinator; *h, h*, triangularis menti; *g, g*, quadratis menti; *i, i*, masseter.

The facial muscles rest decidedly under the influence of conscious volition which allows, to a high degree, the mastery of the involuntary play of the muscles; it is the prerogative of a good education to use this mastery, and at the right times, not by suppressing, in some sort, every involuntary play of the features, but to prevent the animal in man from becoming the ruling expression. To learn this mastery will be imperative, if the early education and manner of life have allowed a distorted mien to become habitual.

For the actor who must give the various personalities he represents another form than that of his own face, and who must do this not merely by mental activity, but by the use of various paints, it is indispensably necessary to know how nature in these various characters fashions the form of the face. We quote therefore some principles from Piderit's "Physiognomy."

4. *Main Elements of Facial Expression.*

The strong-willed, decided man is recognized by his firm glance, while an unsteady glance is peculiar to those who lack confidence in themselves or others, to hunted and guilty men. This glance may, however, result from illness.

If one grasps a representation, the muscles of his eyes will be tense as if grasping some object; if he contrasts different representations, his eyes will be moved as he turns his glance from one to the other, etc.

Intellectual activity may be recognized by a quick, observant glance; while intellectual sluggishness and indifference are betrayed by the empty glance; that is, by a lax, slow movement of the muscles of the eye-ball. The slow and at the same time firm glance, indicates calm deliberation; the quick, and at the same time restless glance, indicates fugitive thought, such as want of consideration, volatility.

A considerable part of the upper edge of the pupil concealed by the lid, denotes intellectual indolence, while raised lids and unveiled pupils are a sign of intellectual activity.

Practical, energetic men are wont to have a near glance; speculators, philosophers, dreamy men let their glance sweep far away. Very enthusiastic men are known by their peculiar and somewhat upturned glance.

Men, who in walking or sitting, bend the head forward, must, in order to gaze before them, draw the pupil high under the lid. This veiled glance is found in people who observe closely, and would yet appear unsympathetic. It is peculiar to distrustful men. If the veiled glance is at the same time firm, it is called lowering (Fig. L.).

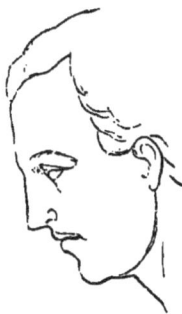

FIG. L.

The tension of the muscles of the forehead is indicated by horizontal folds and uplifted brows. These muscles become tense on the one hand, when the eyes are opened as widely and quickly as possible, and on the other hand, when they are held open as steadily as possible.

The mimic expression, if constantly repeated, becomes part of the physiognomy, and is recognized by horizontal lines in the forehead. If the physiognomical trait is strongly marked, the brows remain drawn upward.

This facial trait of the horizontal line is found:

(*a*) In good-natured men.
(*b*) In curious men.

THE MIMIC ART. 99

(*c*) In men who, by inclination and habit, retain firmly and enduringly the ideas awakened in their souls. I designate these inclinations by the word *contemplativeness.*

Horizontal lines on the forehead, a vacant gaze, and sunken eyelids, denote intellectual indolence, united with good humor or curiosity, or bent for reflection.

The eyebrow muscles draw backward the upper part of the muscle that closes the eyes. The tension of this muscle lays the forehead in perpendicular folds; in like manner the eyebrows become drawn somewhat downward, with their inner ends approaching each other.

We find perpendicular lines:

(*a*) In people who have had much physical suffering.
(*b*) In people who have suffered mentally.
(*c*) In people who have been visited by misfortune.
(*d*) In sensitive, dissatisfied, fretful people.
(*e*) In shortsighted people.

Where the mouth stands more or less open and the under lip retreats more or less, we presuppose an obtuse, muddled intellect (Fig. LI.).

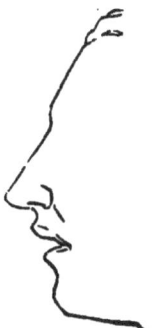

FIG. LI.

Lips more or less knit together denote obstinacy, that is, a mind shut up in its own ideas (Fig. LII.).

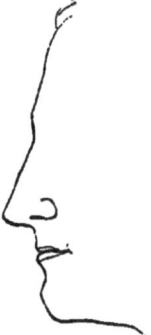

FIG. LII.

We therefore find this trait:
(*a*) In stubborn people.
(*b*) In reliable people.
(*c*) In careful people.
(*d*) In reticent people.
(*e*) In self-seeking, avaricious people.

Lips lying loosely together indicate the contrary; hence susceptibility and frankness.

If one tries some gustatory object (for instance wine) with the organs of taste, he protrudes both lips at the same time, pressing them together and giving the mouth a snout-like form. In this way the cavity of the mouth is widened, while the substance tasted is held fast. This form of the mouth (Fig. LIII.) is therefore found :

(*a*) In gourmands.
(*b*) In critical persons.

If the organ of taste is unpleasantly excited, the arch of the palate is removed as far as possible from the surface of the tongue, the upper lip as far as possible from the under, while the nostrils are raised (Fig. LIV.). We observe the same expression

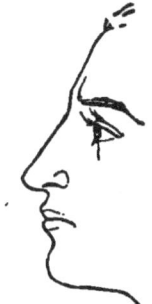

FIG. LIII.

as the sign of an imaginary excitement of the organs of taste; also in a sudden, intense, disagreeable excitement of other organs of sense, or in the excitement of unpleasant ideas. The mimic expression of bitterness will therefore be called forth by inciting ideas whose unpleasant nature is significantly described as "bitter."

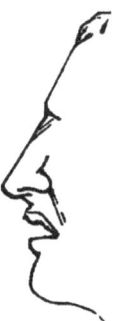

FIG. LIV.

If one is delighted with a pleasant idea, while at the same time agitated by an unpleasant one, the mouth will give slight expression to the bitterness, while the eyes glance upward (Fig. LV.).

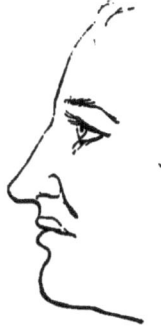

FIG. LV.

A compressed mouth with a bitter expression indicates a stubborn, misanthropic person (Fig. LVI.).

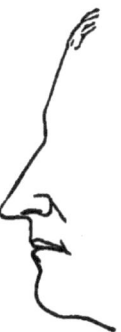

FIG. LVI.

The physical impress of scorn is a deep line under the angle of the lower lips. In this case the chin appears flat, because its flesh is tightly drawn, while the under lip is pressed upward.

The eyelids fall as in drowsiness, while a certain degree of negligent attention is discernible on account of the tension of the muscles of the forehead, whereby the sinking lids are held in place, horizontal lines appearing on the forehead.

GENERAL PHYSIOGNOMICAL REMARKS.

1. *The Cheeks.*

Fleshy cheeks usually indicate a sensitive temperament and susceptibility. If lean and narrow they denote dry humor and a lack of sensuality. Sorrow makes them hollow; coarseness and stupidity imprint them with folds and furrows. Depressions, more or less angular in form, are an infallible sign of envy and jealousy. A line passing from the nostril to the corner of the mouth is very indicative of character; if it is a curve without any variation or wave line, it is an infallible sign of stupidity. It is the same when its end leads, without interruption, along the edge of the upper lip, or lies not far removed from it.

2. *The Lips.*

Fleshy lips indicate sensuality, gourmandism, indolence. Sharply cut lips and those with hard outlines denote unrest and avarice. An elevated upper lip indicates self-importance and coarseness. A thick, protruding lower lip is the sign of a foolishly boastful and withal, intellectually impoverished man. A sullen, lipless mouth, turning upward at the sides, denotes affectation and vanity.

3. *The Chin.*

A protruding chin always denotes something positive; a retreating chin, something negative. A round chin with a dimple, denotes goodness; a small chin indicates timidity, bashfulness; a smooth chin, coldness and dryness of temperament; an angular chin denotes penetration, cleverness and firmness; a pointed chin is a sign of strategy and cunning; a long, broad, fat chin indicates a hard, proud, obstinate, violent character. A chin indicating cleverness must be turned back or cleft in the middle. All that is said here must not serve the dramatic artist as a model whereby alone he is forced to act. It is left for his imagination and talent everywhere to supply the necessary modifications.

CHAPTER III.

GESTURE.

> "Gesture arises from the passion it is to represent. It is an arrow winged by the soul; it must have speedy effect and reach the goal to which the cord of sensation hurries it on. After we are instructed in the principles of our art, let us follow the impulses of our souls. If our sensations are keen, they cannot mislead us."—NOVERRE'S LETTERS.

When fully grounded in the plastic of the human limbs, gesture comes almost without effort; it arises always from inward emotion, and one incapable of such emotion, may study whole volumes upon gesture without deriving any special benefit from them.

THE SINGLE LIMBS IN RELATION TO GESTURE.

Of all members of the body, the arms and hands are most active in gesture. Before laying down fundamental rules, we will briefly consider the head as a whole, and for this purpose, borrow something from "The Symbolical in the Human Form," by Carus.

1. The Head.

In bending the head forward, it is the forehead, the symbol of intelligence, which sinks or falls, and thus necessarily gives recognition of a truth outwardly presented, such as assent; further, assent to another's opinion, also submission to another's understanding, and finally, weariness,—a yielding up of conscious intellectual mastery, a transition into sleep. At the same time it happens that the intellectual region, that is the region of the brain, inclines forward,— a decided symbol of mental sympathy and assent.

The opposite movement, the uplifting of the forehead, must

indicate the reverse. Every such uplifting elevates the seat of intelligence above all outside of it, and all sympathy of feeling is expressed by a backward inclination of the head. Hence it happens that a medium mood of the soul, removed alike from assent and dissent, from humiliation and scorn, can find outward expression only in the calm uplifting of the head. It is also evident which of these three tendencies or soul-moods in the life of man is uppermost, by the carriage of the head which will infallibly express one or the other; for instance, the head thrown backward will express pride and vanity, the head bent forward, mildness, submission, condescension and subjection; while calmness and quiet self-persistence will find expression in a simple, but firm and upright carriage of the head.

To the three movements above mentioned may be added that emphatic throwing back of the head which, in every case, points to the prevailing tendency of the *wishful* and craving soul, symbolically indicated by the region of the back head. Every inordinately violent exertion of energy, all strong desires make the hind part of the head the prevailing pole of the head movement and draw it backward.

A weak sideward inclination of the head is indicative of exhaustion and mental over-exertion; a more or less forward inclination denotes sorrow, depression and discouragement. If the sideward movement is more decided, doubt is expressed; doubt with astonishment by a sort of swaying motion from left to right. A mere turning to the right or left denotes dissatisfaction, opposition or aversion. If, at the same time, the head is bent backward or uplifted, it is characterized as a looking over the shoulder, a gesture of scorn or of impudent challenge. The mere sideward turning to and fro is denial; if this happens several times in quick, abrupt succession, to the right and left, it is shaking the head and thus the denial or displeasure is emphasized or finds expression in impatience, dejection or displeasure. A quiet shaking of the head is a sign of doubt upon some matter, or certain sort of surprise. Shoving forward the head with an elevation of the chin, is a sign of curiosity, and indicates listening ; hence we find this movement in individuals who are caught listening.

2. *The Arms and Hands in General.*

Quintilian says of the use of the hands :

"While the other limbs assist the speaker, the hands, I dare affirm, speak themselves. For do we not demand, promise, call, dismiss, threaten, entreat, abhor, fear, ask, deny with them? Do we not indicate joy, sadness, doubt, acknowledgement, remorse, measure, multitude, number and time with them? Do they not arouse courage? Do they not mourn, repel, consent? Do they not express admiration and shame? This is the language which in the great diversity of tongues among all races and peoples, I have in common with all men."

If Quintilian, who wrote only for orators, speaks thus of the hand, of what importance must it be in the representation of the whole man !

Some animals have horns ; others have hoofs, teeth, claws, talons, spurs and beaks ; man has nothing of the sort ; he is placed weak and defenseless in the world, but the hand aside from its practical use, gives him compensation for all this.

It is impossible to give, it would be absurd to attempt to give all the movements of which the head and arm are capable. In accordance with the purpose of our book we present only fundamental rules.

Physical Gymnastics have taught us the movements of which the arm is capable ; we now consider briefly their significance in acting.

The arms may hang quietly at the side, but in this posture they express no mental emotion. A crossing of the arms over the breast indicates investigation ; a crossing of them behind the back indicates attention merely. In the former case the body bends forward ; in the latter, backward. In acting, the hand is the all-important member. It stands in the same controlling relation to the upper and lower arm that the eye or mouth has to other parts of the face.

The hand is important to the actor, not only on account of its general movements, but also from the fact that the fingers enable it to open or close with various degrees of force.

Thus a hand slightly closed denotes mildness; while in the semblance of defiance or contempt, the closed fist and the inner side of the arm are turned toward the one threatened. Real rage turns the inner side of the arm and the clinched fist toward him.

Furthermore, the fingers of the hand and their movements are of great import in acting. The thumb must be called the clinching finger, since it gives its character of defiance to the clinched hand. It is at the same time the most technical finger among the five, and the strongest. It also serves for mental expression, as, for instance, (Fig. LVII.) in the scorn evident of what is past

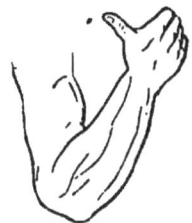

Fig. LVII.

or not present. The finger next the thumb is aptly called the index, or demonstrative finger. It points always in a noble way, and contempt is foreign to it. Its office is pure demonstration, it serves as an expression of the reason rather than the sensibilities. Place, things, time and persons, are pointed out by it. (Fig. LVIII.)

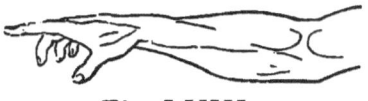

Fig. LVIII.

Next to the index finger stands the third, the so-called middle finger, the longest. In acting, it should be called the wishing finger. We observe how greedy for an object really at hand is he who points to it with this finger. (Fig. LIX.) The finger next

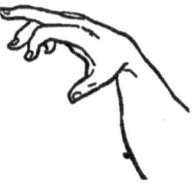

Fig. LIX.

to this is called the fourth. It might be named the feeling and testing finger. If one would scratch the chin or rub the eyes gently, he uses this finger. Those born blind teach themselves at first only by feeling with the index finger. The last finger is called the fifth or little finger. The actor might call it the belittling finger, for it expresses belittlement in a noble or ironic sense. One need only recall how naturally he touches the tip of the little finger with the thumb to indicate the *little*.

In works on German art dating from the middle ages, we seldom see a hand in true, noble repose. The mediæval Germans, for the most part, delineated the hand with its fingers lying close together, indicative of effort; or they gave the hand a genuine expression. In the statues of ancient Greece, on the contrary, the repose of the hand is masterly. The fingers are bent, but not obtrusively, the index finger least of all. Hence on to the little finger the curvature increases as if to show the capability of the hand in demonstration. (Fig. LX). The fingers are not

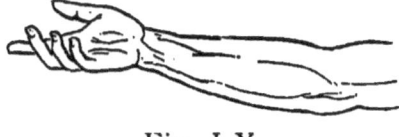

Fig. LX.

pressed together, they are separated, but not so much that the separation seems forced.

3. Main Principles of the Position of the Hand in Acting.

This portion of our work is founded upon Ling's book, adapted by Hugo Rothstein. He divides the various positions of the hand into the following groups :

(*a*) Hand flat and horizontal with inner palm upward, with under arm held up, or the whole arm extended or held forward, indicates offering, explanation, salutation. In grasping hands in salutation, naturally the hand of him who salutes is offered, while that of the other only grasps it, and therefore takes the inverted position.

(*b*) Hand flat and horizontal with inner palm downward is the gesture of protection, guardianship, blessing, confirmation, of irrevocable decision and conclusion ; also the gesture commanding repose and silence. Alternating with (*a*) it indicates gazing around, contemplation.

(*c*) Hand vertical with inner palm reversed, lower arm drawn forward, the whole arm more or less elevated, is a sympathetic gesture, for beckoning, for presentation, for well-meant or earnest meaning, for reproach, etc. ; also a gesture of contemplative thought, intuition, etc.

(*d*) Hand vertical with inner palm forward, with under arm raised or fully extended is antipathetic, evasive, repellent, expressive of abhorrence, fear, horror ; with the arm raised high, the utmost horror.

(*e*) Hand with thumb downward and inner palm outward ; with arm more or less extended, or united with a side movement of the same is repellent, setting aside, displacing, casting out, not wishing to know of something ; it is also the gesture of contempt, etc.

(*f*) Hand with thumb upward and inner palm inward ; lower arm still raised forward, with elbows against the body, or the whole arm extended more or less, is separating, sundering, discriminating, rending.

These six main positions of the hand are taken with one hand or with both together. In the first case the other hand remains passive, or makes a complementary gesture, but in other cases both hands unite by

(*g*) Laying the inner palms together with the hands horizontal and usually one crossed over the other, rarely with a quiet bearing, but with constant beating of the upper against the lower hand ; commanding repose or silence, but used, also, for the liveliest clapping in applause ; or both hands with their length line horizontal, their cross line vertical, and thumbs upward wedge-shaped as if to separate something, a position of the hand quite habitual with preachers and schoolmasters. Joined with clapping this is a gesture of real or malicious joy ; or both hands vertical, and usually on a level with the breast, for persistent entreaty as well as for prayer, in which case the fingers lie tensely one against the other or are entwined.

(*h*) The hands folded crosswise, inner palm upon inner palm, but with locked thumbs and fingers, denotes a humble, reverent bearing sometimes used in prayer.

(*i*) Laying of the back of one hand upon the palm of the other, or both inner palms turned upward, both hands somewhat bent, the arms pendent, either before or behind or both inner palms downward, and the arm hanging stiffly in front, denotes passiveness, comfort, etc. In certain sorts of admiration, also in involuntary admiration, the arms are elevated and brought forward. This manner of holding the hands also expresses a feeble degree of despair, and the whole gesture is something like that of wringing the hands.

(*j*) Folding the hands with the fingers interlaced, if the fingers only twine loosely—this manner of holding the hands with the arms at the same time hanging laxly, indicates nothing more than repose or comfort, otherwise a self-contained nature, introspection, devotion, and similar mental moods, the deeper and more ardent the latter, so much the nearer do the inner palms approach ; they even unite in an intense pressure, in which case both folded hands are carried to the breast, and more or less pressed against it. Besides, this folding of the hands serves for a gesture of earnest entreaty.

(*k*) Wringing the hands, a gesture difficult to describe, because it is movable and changeable so far as the hands are concerned. The hands certainly remain in contact, still not in a decided grasp. The fingers meantime are now closed, now folded, the arms in restless movement, now bent, now extended, now raised, now lowered, etc. This gesture naturally occurs only in very deep and powerful excitement, in the most profound agony and despair.

4. *The Torso.*

In Physical Gymnastics we have learned the torso's capability for movement, in turning and bending forward, backward and sideward. What significance have these in acting?

An easy, but still firm and erect carriage of the torso, indicates self-esteem and dignity.

Bending forward always expresses a sympathy for the object toward which the torso inclines ; bending backward expresses antipathy. The first, therefore, denotes affection, confidence, readiness to assist, benevolence, friendliness, etc. ; the second, aversion, distrust, hatred, etc.

A drawing sideward, as if turning away from something, expresses disregard, distrust, scorn ; and an entire turning, in which naturally the foot takes part, expresses these sentiments in the highest degree.

In the side movement as if turning toward something, there lies, in fact, a certain degree of sympathy ; but if the foot does not take part in the movement, there is here a sort of disregard and indifference.

To draw back the shoulders with the chest arched, indicates

courage, boldness and especially self-confidence. This attitude strongly marked, denotes haughtiness, arrogance and scorn.

Drawing forward the shoulders with the consequent drawing in of the chest, is the sign of anguish, fear, despondency, etc.

A drawing downward of the shoulders occurs mostly in sudden terror. Connected with the drawing of them upward produces the gesture of shrugging.

5. *The Legs and Feet.*

The action of the legs and feet in mere progression, has been accurately described in "The Mechanism of the Walking Apparatus." Aside from their office in walking the legs and feet have another office : The support and carriage of the torso in all positions. Even regarding them only as supporters, we find them not entirely passive in gesture. However, they perform their destined office under all circumstances, even if the body is not for the moment in motion. If the gesture of standing is complete the position of the feet must show exactly whether the gesture indicates progression or not.

In all the gestures carried out in standing in which the feet take an active share, one of the feet must always sustain the body, while the other assumes the motion.

Hence, according to Rothstein, arises the designation of one foot as the standing, the other the acting foot. There are but few cases where this distinction does not enter, and both feet alike sustain the body ; these are the stiff, arbitrary position of the soldier before his superior, and that of the servant before his master. Here the heels are close together, or one is close against the inner edge of the other foot, the knees being tense. This position, although the body is sustained by both feet, is by no means one of repose ; it is an arduous one, and expresses subordination, obedience ; a strict inward sense of the commands and charges to be given, as well as a forced, stiff manner ; hence only for brief moments can it remain the attitude of voluntary respect and obedience. As soon as this forced subordination grows somewhat lax, one foot loosens a little and its knee bends slightly, while the line of gravity passes more and more to the other foot. At this first effort of the one foot for freedom, the relations of standing and acting foot alternate. In acting, the alternation of the standing foot must be so managed that the original standing-place may be retained by the actor.

From such transpositions of the feet arise those various positions in which the body sometimes remains only for a moment, but often for a greater or less length of time. The main forms are: The standing position, the walking, stepping and side position, and the thrust position. The striding or walking position expresses, as a rule, a tendency to move forward. Setting the foot forward indicates meeting, stepping together, reception, offering, etc. Setting back the foot indicates withdrawal, flinching, fleeing, renunciation, etc. Assuming the side position may also indicate progression, but only in the sense of avoidance or withdrawal. This attends very emphatically, for instance the gesture of contempt. The thrust position, results usually from a sudden and violent excitement, and for the most part, accompanies only very animated action. As taken backward or forward and according to the bearing of the upper body and the upper extremities, it may express very different things. For instance, a setting back of the foot, and bending back of the upper part of the body, is the gesture of the highest sort of horror.

We must here briefly distinguish the different angles of the positions of the feet. The outward rectangular position is the normal one ; the obtuse angle is forced, does not present sufficient firmness, reminds one of the dancing master, indicates an affected manner (affectation). The acute angle leads to the inward position, and expresses helplessness, awkwardness, stupidity, coarseness, etc. Each of the aforesaid foot positions can be carried out only by the help and support of the legs, consequently it relates to these also.

6. *Walking in Acting.*

We have learned to understand the natural gait as a mere onward movement as well as in its æsthetic sense ; but something remains to be added in regard to the walk in acting.

Whether the walk is for the dramatic representation of given characters or for special intellectual excitement, several shades and modulations enter into the movement.

It is evident that, for instance, joy and pleasure bring with them a perceptibly increased swiftness of movement, while with sorrow and melancholy, there would be a perceptible decrease. Exalted moods and passions require an increased swiftness. Courage and decision show a secure, firm tread ; cowardice, a weak, wavering gait, a slow, or at least, very moderate *tempo*. In anguish and horror, the gait is tottering ; in courage and fury, tempestuous. Hypocrisy and treachery sneak along ; silliness and vanity move with short, tripping steps and feet much turned outward ; phlegm (indifference) and idleness have a slow and slipping or rather slouching gait ; scorn a stamping gait, etc.

In general, it may be said that the further a man's special character departs from the ideal of true manhood, the greater his moral faults and weaknesses, so much wider become his departures from the normal gait, from the bounds required by grace and dignity, and so much the more decidedly will his gait indicate one fault or the other, or the several forms of fault.

Although the structure of our walking apparatus tends naturally to going forward, and this is the normal method of walking, it also admits of walking backward. If, for instance, one would withdraw from a person to whom reverence is due, decorum demands that this take place with single, backward steps, with the face fixed upon the revered person ; then the full turn for walking forward is made. Neglect of this rule renders one liable to the reproach of ill-breeding, disrespect and irreverence. Also, in great surprise, in astonishment, horror, etc., one walks backward some steps.

Walking forward usually takes place in a direct line, but mental or outside motives often require a circuitous direction. If, for instance, two persons in walking meet upon one line, one of them must step aside ; common politeness demands that in two persons of the same station, both should do this ; but in meeting an honored personage, we leave the path free for him. In like manner, the gentleman steps aside for the lady, the young for the old.

Among the mental motives which lead to walking in curved lines, are suspicion, embarrassment, espionage, anxiety, despair, etc.

In regard to going up to a person which is to be distinguished from a mere meeting, no decided rules can be given, since many local conditions intervene. But this much may be said : In approaching a person of higher rank, the walk, if before rapid, must grow slower and more dignified, and a pause occur at least two steps distant from him ; in the case of a prince, three steps. (See Parts Fourth and Seventh.)

An important characteristic in walking in common life and far more so upon the stage, is the ability to measure with certainty the distance. A firm, clear-sighted individual knows how many steps he must take to reach his goal, whether the steps be long or short. Undecided characters never know this, and, therefore, come hastening too near the object or not near enough, or make several missteps. An actor should be able to measure with bandaged eyes the dimensions of the stage in all directions, and let his gait be measured by circumstances. We often notice the absurd gait of one who hands a letter, or perhaps has to take some trifling thing upon the stage. Often in such cases servants approach too near their masters, or pause too far away, so that the master is obliged to come to meet them. Comic actors well know how to raise a laugh in this way.

7. Characteristic Tokens of Several Kinds of Gait.

The heavy gait is thus characterized by Harless : At the

moment when the centre of gravity falls over the axis of the middle of the foot, the swinging foot has already set its heel on the floor, near that point. One walks in this manner after severe illness, in bearing heavy burdens carefully over a smooth surface, especially when the nature of the ground or the muscular strength at command advises caution. The nearer the heel of the forward foot is set near the ball of the backward foot, so much the more constrained will be the gait. This gait may be slow or rapid as the line of gravity approaches nearer the foremost foot. It indicates a sort of insecurity, anxiety or cautiousness; and is, therefore, often employed by elderly people or invalids, or for walking in the twilight. The space in which the body rests only on one leg will, for this reason, be shortened as much as possible.

The shuffling gait upon the soles of the feet is thus described: The hindmost foot does not lift its ball from the floor before the forward foot resumes its standing position. We find this gait among the blind, in groping and creeping. In the latter, we also find walking on tip-toe, where the body is usually bent somewhat forward.

The Swaying Gait.—This arises less from bending the knee than from turning the hip. We find it united with a heavy step in fleshy people, in bearing upon the head heavy burdens or objects liable to break, in walking upon stilts, in the heavy stage step in caricature.

Akin to this is a gait in which the sole of the foot is considered immovable, and, therefore, at every step falls with its whole surface on the ground. In this gait, the steps are very short, and the line of gravity always falls upon the heel of the foremost foot. This is the "Turkish gait" of the stage.

The Dignified Gait.—In this gait the upper body which stands erect, with knees more or less stiff, seems to be drawn out and elongated from the hips. The time during which both feet touch the floor, is therefore the longest. Here the more or less decides infinitely much. An inch more and we see a caricature.

If, in this gait, the toes are set down first and too soon the result is

The Dancing-master Step.—This step arises from swaying the body sideways and is, consequently, insecure. The groping gait is the same, and the standing foot is more or less bent from the knee.

THE LIMBS IN HARMONIOUS ACTION.

1. The Divisions of Gesture.

Ling divides the various gestures of which man is capable into five classes:

(*a*) Expressive,
(*b*) Delineative,
(*c*) Interpretative,
(*d*) Imitative and
(*e*) Conventional.

(*a*) *Expressive gestures* we call those which characterize only individual mental states. To embody such gestures requires a lively fancy and a fine gift of observation. If the actor is devoid of the latter, he will give us the expression of his own emotions, but not those of various individuals. Here the actor must guard carefully against exaggerations; one step too far, and the sublime becomes ridiculous. Rules cannot be given for this first class of gestures. A lively fancy, a cultivated intellect, a fine tact always strike the right medium.

The portrayal of anger and despair presents the most difficulties to the actor; his own excitability is apt to take away his presence of mind and carry him beyond the limits of the beautiful.

(*b*) *Delineative gestures* are those which embody the idea of outward objects or their moods and peculiarities. If, for instance, one would materialize the surging of the sea, the contours of a house, a line, a cross, the fusion of two bodies, etc., he helps the words by the aid of an outlining, depicting gesture. In this sort of gestures, the actor must guard against overacting, against seeking to depict everything. In this way he falls irretrievably into the ridiculous.

The fundamental rule here is: Always grasp the whole, but outline main ideas only, and especially avoid every delineative gesture which does not stand in intimate connection with one's own feelings.

(*c*) *Interpretative gestures* are distinguished from delineative ones in that they only express symbolically the common attributes of space, time and strength. For instance: Height, depth, nearness, width, haste, strength, weakness, multitude, procrastination, etc.

(*d*) *Imitative gestures* are strict imitations of the ways of another without entering into his intellectual life and to act accordingly. Here, also, the right medium must be strictly observed. According to Ling imitative gestures are also delineative ones. "Here is the same distinction we make in technical drawing, drawing after models as copying, or from nature according to our own ideas or fancy. The copyist is strictly bound to his model, and the more closely his copy represents the model with all its peculiarities, and even its faults, the better it is."

(*e*) *Conventional gestures* are those which are executed by tacit consent or custom. To this class belong the ceremonies of entire corporations, as well as those individual ones which must always be learned from life, and to enumerate which is impossible. The dramatic expression will be modified by age, temperament, habit, national and popular customs.

To elucidate this subject further would be foreign to the purpose of this book. We only append Rothstein's words in regard to modifications that belong to different periods of life:

"The most casual observer cannot fail to perceive how much these main steps must be modified by age. The gestures of youth are animated, its manner restless. The youthful mind easily excited, but usually ingenuous, will express itself in its own untrammeled way if not restrained by outside influences, or toned down by education. The old man expresses himself with very few gestures, dwelling longer upon passages, and in general with measured dignity. He lives more inwardly, is without lively emotions, and displays but little feeling. In middle life, the imitative movements are strong, decided, expressive, but more moderate than in youth. The mature man controls his gestures, often represses them, and not seldom affects reserve, even to extreme dissimulation. He weighs his position in life, his circumstances and surroundings, and conforms his actions to them."

It is self-evident that the manner of gesture must be in accord with the costume and age to which the piece belongs. It would, for instance, be entirely wrong to give an antique figure the step and movement of a person of the time of Louis XIV. or vice versa. The same distinction must be made between a figure of that time and a modern one.

We will return to the above at the description of Compliments.

2. The Fundamental Rules for Correct Action of the Limbs in Gesture are as follows:

(*a*) Every gesture must render simply, truthfully, but decidedly what it has to express. This law applies to the gesture of the doubtful as well as to that of the certain. In the former case, the very doubt must be decidedly expressed. Hence it follows:

(*b*) That every movement not proceeding from the mass of emotions to be portrayed, must be unavailing. Let the gesture be ever so beautiful, if it does not obey this law, it will become unsightly.

(*c*) The play of the features must always precede the gesture; but in depicting very excited mental moods, the gesture often precedes the words. As a rule, it accompanies the text, and coincides with it. If the text demands that a gesture should end the words, it follows upon them.

(*d*) Gesture must not end voluntarily while speech still goes on; it must accompany the words to the end; and as in acting there is no pause, the actor, after his speech is ended, must reflect in his own features, in his eye at least, that which the other speaks. Here most actors fail. The body, the face is animated only while they are speaking ; when done speaking they fall into a physical as well as mental inactivity, which destroys all harmony. Hence dumb play is the most difficult of all. Here the true artist is manifest.

(*e*) Great care must be taken that the movements of the limbs be not exaggerated. To use a military simile, the actor must not shoot with cannon when small shot will answer.

We have already laid down the fundamental law for arm-movements. "As few movements as possible," we repeat here in regard to all gesture. The sins against this law are many and surprising. We give a few instances:—The head should be turned gracefully and quickly to one side. Instead of this, the whole body is turned often with constant shifting of the feet. The whole hand and even the arm, is used to designate what could be pointed out by the little finger.

Many examples might be given. These two will illustrate our meaning. How is it possible to indicate an ascending scale in passion by gesture, if we begin with the strongest?

(*f*) *All* the limbs must unite in one gesture, and single limbs must not be entirely in repose, while the others express something. We add in order not to be misunderstood : All the limbs should not share alike in one gesture, but they must all express the intention of this gesture ; that is, the actor must not make a decided gesture with his hand, while his feet are wholly in repose ; he must not decidedly indicate an object with one hand and the upper part of the body bent forward, while the other hand, as if not belonging to this body, hangs limp and passive at the side. A lively, but restrained imagination, a gymnastically trained body will observe the right mean.

(*g*) Gestures must not come close together ; they must be developed from one another. Hence, there must be no abruptness in gesture, if it is not required for expression. If, for instance, we would express joy, and then immediately after it, horror, these gestures must by a rightly defined transition, proceed from one another; that is, the mind must retain a part, be it ever so small, of the former mood, before the new one can be fully developed. This part of acting is the most difficult of arts; its right practice is the stamp of perfection.

(*h*) The stage walk must conform exactly to the character represented, as well while playing as when appearing on the stage and leaving it. We often see the actor enter with his usual gait, while the play requires that of the rôle. In leaving he also falls back into his own gait. This destroys that illusion which is the object of all acting.

Entrance upon and exit from the stage are alike difficult. Because the actor seldom speaks upon his entrance he forgets his imitative character and remembers it only when his words begin, which is false. Here let it be remarked that many actors lay little stress upon the number of steps they take in presence of the audience; in this way they mar the characterization. The law of beauty demands that no steps be taken except those required by the situation. Here also we must lay down the fundamental law as in arm-movements : " As few as possible." Repose is the main thing in a picture. An actor shows little culture, if in representing a crowned head, he finds no way to express his dignity save in striding around the stage.

(*i*) It is self-evident that in acting the player never forces himself to the front unless the character or the situation demand it, and yet so many unpardonable blunders of this kind happen, that we must say a few words in regard to them. If the actor remains true to the character and situation, exaggeration is impossible ; but we often see an actor so exert himself to make a great deal out of a minor part, that we turn from him in aversion. The actor must not go an inch beyond his rôle, otherwise he will destroy its effect and incur the reproach of presumption, vanity and an inordinate desire for applause. The true actor, when upon the stage, regards himself as but a co-worker for the attainment of a common goal.

Just as reprehensible is the manner of some modern virtuosos, who either cut out the minor rôles of a piece, or shorten them so that nothing of the author's work remains but a parade rôle, which is sure to be the one most applauded by the public, while the co-actors, whose every chance for effect is cut off, sink in its estimation as artists. This sort of clap-trap arising from a miserable vanity or desire for speculation, has had its day, thank heaven! Let us hope that its end is near.

3. *Of the Use of the Left and Right Hand.*

My pupils have often put to me the question: "What is your opinion on the use of the right and left hand? Do you deem the more frequent use of the right hand an act induced by habit or by inner, organic causes?" These are questions that require no answer in our book, still we have to point out how the actor must use them.

Both arms and hands must be educated alike in order that the left may be used at the left, the right at the right side. No movement must take place with the right hand to the left side and vice versa. To allow only the slightest movement to the left hand while the whole burden of motion falls upon the right hand, betrays the untrained actor. And still, we find this fault in distinguished actors. Circumstances arise upon the stage, when, as in daily life, the right hand only must be used, as in the oath, the shaking of hands, etc. All this whether one stands to the left or right on the stage must be executed with the right hand; but if an occasion arises when either may be used, in the movement to the left, it must always be the left hand that is taken; in that to the right, always the right hand. Here, for example, belongs the kiss of the hand. If the lady stands upon the gentleman's left he may be easily led to take her hand in his right instead of his left hand; but this would look awkward. (See

Handkiss). Just so, if one would hand or pass something from or to the left side, he all too readily employs the right hand. This is entirely wrong.

If in sitting at table one has to serve wine to the right and left (although serving usually takes place with the right hand), he must reverse our rule and serve to left with the right and to right with the left hand, since it is awkward to hold the wine-bottle in such a way that the nails of the hand are turned upward, or to turn around so much that one's back is to one's neighbor.

It is absolutely necessary in daily life, as upon the stage, that the hands be trained in like manner. If in daily life we have not always a public before us, we have one around us in society, and it is both awkward and discourteous, if when sitting with the left side to the table and with the body inclined forward, we take from it a cup of tea, or whatever else it may be, with the right hand. This always shows a lack of *tournure*.

4. *Greeting, Prayer, Oath.*

The expressions and signs in salutation, vary greatly among different nations. That kind feeling inborn in every man, as well as its expressions and tokens embodied in the salutation, are more or less diversified according to the degree of his culture, his religious and political ideas, his nationality, race, position and social rank. Thus the manner of greeting indicates, in some sort, the elementary character of a people, a tribe, and, in many respects, a single individual.

The Orientals always have been and still remain far more voluble and ceremonious in their manner of salutation than the Occidentals. Among all Asiatic people it is the custom to prostrate one's self in token of utter subjection, while serfdom in Europe required this only partially and incidentally. Until very recently, Asiatic subjects addressed their kings only kneeling or prostrate in the dust, regarding them as supernatural beings. This manner of salutation first came in vogue among the Romans, under the reign of Diocletian, (about A. D. 300). The custom in Europe may be regarded as an after-growth, respect and submission having been until quite recently expressed merely by kneeling, a practice still common in Russia.

5. Salutations of the Hebrews.

(*a*) *Benediction.*— Divine service was ended by the priestly benediction with extended hands and bowed form : " The Lord bless thee and keep thee," etc. The priest who gave the benediction, covered his face with both hands. (Fig. LXI.)

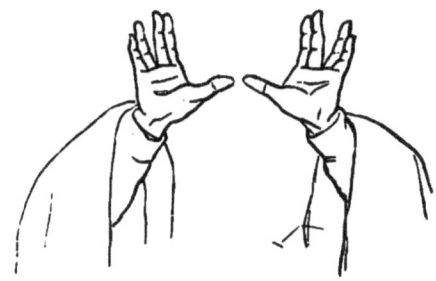

FIG. LXI.

For the better understanding of the position of the fingers the engraver has shown the hands in an upright position. They must, however, be held bent forward though directly covering the face.

(*b*) *The Civil Greeting.*—Not to return a salutation was considered the height of ill-breeding. It was, however, the custom not to salute those mourning or fasting,—a custom still in vogue. Distinguished persons must be greeted, however, but if they were fasting or in sorrow, they need return no answer.

In coming and going, as well as in meeting, the lower bowed before the higher, repeated his obeisance, bowed more profoundly according to the rank of the person greeted, sometimes falling upon the earth. People also fell upon one another's necks and exchanged kisses. The kiss was a token of mutual good wishes, also a sign of reverence and homage. It was given upon arrival, at meeting and parting. The mouth or beard was grasped by the hand, and kissed. Toward princes, the kiss was a sign of homage. As such, it was imprinted upon the hand or knee.

The Hebrew never uncovered the head in greeting high or low. In like manner he prayed — prays to this day — with covered head. It was a shame for women to uncover the head. The head of the woman found guilty of adultery was violently bared by the priest.

The uncovering of the head as now practiced in Europe to express reverence, respect, good will, came after the promulgation of Christianity, but became with higher culture, a symbol of salutation among men. (Women never uncover the head in greetings). Notwithstanding the Hebrew custom of covering the head in sacrifice or prayer, the apostle Paul forbade it. And so it happened that among later Christians, it became a fashion to uncover the head to exalted persons in token of reverence or kind wishes.

(*c*) *Position in Prayer.*— The Hebrew who prays, stands with his face to the east, his form erect, his feet together, his hands folded across his breast, or their palms folded and in this way raised to heaven. He retains this attitude during his whole prayer. Whenever the name of God occurs in his prayer, he bows more or less profoundly. The Hebrew never prays kneeling; but in the temple, the whole congregation fall on their knees, as soon as the name of God is uttered. When the prayer ends the suppliant takes a few steps backward to denote this. Naturally this happens only in long prayers.

(*d*) *The Oath.*—In the oath the Hebrew raised his right hand to heaven.

6. *The Moslem Salutation.*

(*a*) *Prayer.*— The Mussulman prays like the Hebrew with covered head. The one who prays, stands with his face toward Mecca, lifts both hands to his face, touches the tips of the ear with the end of his thumb, and says: "God is very great!"

Then he begins his prayer, now standing, now kneeling, now with nose and forehead touching the floor.

If he prays kneeling, he sits upon his heels, his hands with outspread fingers, resting upon the thigh or above the knee; sometimes he rises and makes low reverences. The Mussulman prays so assiduously that if in journeying he comes to water, he washes his hands and then spreads out a rug and prays.

If he prays standing and does not know in what direction Mecca lies, he keeps turning around during prayer.

In taking an oath, the Turk raises one or all the fingers of the right hand.

(*b*) *The Citizen's Greeting.*—The usual salutation in meeting is, "Peace be with you!" The answer is the same. This is called the *selam*.

Among highly-bred people it is the custom for him who first salutes, as well as for him who returns the salutation, to lay the right hand upon the heart, or in rare instances to touch his lips, then his forehead or turban with the same hand. This is called the *tejmineh*, and is the most respectful manner of greeting, the one especially used in intercourse with distinguished people.

Among the Moslems, Persians and Egyptians, if people of lower rank meet those of a higher, the *selam* is seldom uttered; it is expressed symbolically by touching the heart, the seat of emotion, with the hand, bowing in deepest humility and then touching the earth, lips and forehead with the hand. It is quite usual among the Moslems for the one who salutes to place both hands on the turban.

There is also a prevalent custom of kissing the hand, usually upon the wrist or palm, and then laying it on the forehead to express peculiar respect, submission and humility. The deepest submission is shown by kissing the foot instead of the hand. The son kisses the hand of his father, the woman that of her husband, the slave and also the freed servant that of the master. A great man's slaves or servants kiss their master's sleeve or the hem of his garment.

Friends salute by each placing his right hand in that of the other; then each kisses his own hand, carries it to his lips or forehead, or merely lays it on his heart without kissing it.

After long separation, they embrace or fall upon each other's necks and kiss, first upon the right then upon the left cheek or the neck. The head is never uncovered in salutation.

The laughable custom of bowing in supposed Oriental fashion upon the stage with hands crossed upon the breast, should give place to the true method.

(c) *At Visits.*— Upon entering the room in which the master of the house sits, one utters the *selam*. The host returns the salutation. If the visitor is of lower rank, the master of the house remains sitting; if of the same rank, he makes a slight movement as if to rise. If he stands higher in office, religious or scientific repute, the host rises and approaches, according to rank, one or more steps to the middle of the room, to the door, to the passage between the chamber and the court, or into the court itself.

If the visitor stands higher or not lower than the master of the house, he receives a pipe from the latter; in other cases he is served by his slaves. A cup of coffee is then set near each. While the visitor takes the coffee with or without a pipe, he salutes the host with the *tejmineh*, which is returned. The same happens when he gives back the cup to the servant. In the same manner the host salutes the guest every time he receives his cup and hands it back, in case he is not far below him in rank.

If the visitor is of higher rank, the host will accompany him to the stairs or door.

7. *Chinese Salutations.*

While we find dignified reverences among the Hebrews and

Moslems, we see among the Chinese more bowing than obeisances, quick successions of them indeed with much clasping of hands.

Of all Oriental peoples, the Chinese are the only ones who offer salutation with bared head like the Europeans, but this is only before magistrates and when one wears a broad-brimmed straw hat. A silent, respectful attitude is indispensable in presence of an officer, who himself gazes down in scorn. This law of etiquette must be strictly observed. Before exalted personages it is the custom to bow profoundly, to even prostrate one's self upon the earth.

The Chinese honor the gods whose statues are in people's houses, by prostration before them. Before the emperor, one prostrates himself, and touches the floor nine times with his forehead.

Upon entering and leaving a court of justice, subalterns make a low bow to the officers.

8. *Hindoos, Greeks and Romans.*

The Hindoo salutation consists in touching the forehead and bowing the head to the earth. In Sumatra and other East India islands, it consists in prostrating one's self on the ground or placing the foot of the person saluted upon one's head.

The Greeks, in praying and taking oaths, raised both arms and hands, with the inner palms together, the little fingers turned outward.

The Romans likewise raised both arms, but with this difference: The inner palms were outward and still turned upward by a backward movement of the wrist. In both cases the fingers must be neither clasped nor apart, but maintain their natural position.

It was an old Greek and Roman custom to greet the coming and departing guest with a shake of the hand, always giving the right hand. Among all ancient peoples the right hand was sacred. Blood relatives and intimate friends did not give the hand only; they embraced and kissed each other.

It was the Roman custom to kiss not the lips only, but the right hand. Among the ancients there was a sort of kiss in which boys grasped both ears of their parents and other relatives with both hands, and thus kissed. Lovers also kissed in this way.

The Romans in all things showed greater honor to rulers than to private individuals. When rulers came and went, all present rose from their seats. In meeting them the head was uncovered.

9. Salutation, Oath and Prayer of Modern Times According to the European Fashion among Civilized People.

The uncovering of the head is a general custom. Once practiced only in presence of people of high rank, it has been in vogue as a common salutation since the seventeenth century.

The Russians, upon Easterday, salute with a kiss on the forehead. In Poland the peasant greets the priest with a kiss on the hand; the higher classes grasp the hand, but instead of kissing it, they still retain it, and kiss the priest's shoulder.

The greeting of the present day consists in removing the hat with gentlemen; in a slight bow with ladies.

The *rococo* time ordained that in removing the hat and placing it on the head, no bow should be made, but the hand perform the whole business. Modern custom demands that the removal of the hat be accompanied with a slight bow and turn of the head toward the one saluted. The hat must always be grasped with the hand opposite the glance, and remain off the head until one is quite beyond the line of the person greeted. The hand must meantime hold the hat in such a way that its inside is not turned toward the one saluted, but toward one's self.

Military salutations are subject to certain rules, and demand a special study foreign to the purpose of our book.

Salutation in a room takes place by a bow more or less profound according to the rank of the person saluted. This subject is further treated under the head of "Compliment."

The Oath of Christian people is taken by men with an uplifting of the right arm and holding up of the three fingers from the thumb, while the last two are turned inward. The fingers held up must not be in close contact but retain their natural position. Women and priests place the three fingers only on the left side of the heart.

Prayer is made by Catholics mostly while kneeling ; by Protestants standing with bowed heads and clasped hands.

It is self-evident that all rules given under the heads, Salutation, Prayer and Oaths must not be slavishly imitated upon the stage ; but if the actor would grasp the various characteristics, he can do so only by a full knowledge of their use. It is left to his fine tact to appropriate what is necessary and proper for the serious as well as the comic drama.

VARIOUS FAULTY GESTURES AND THEIR CORRECTION.

1. Drinking.

If the actor has a full glass in his hand, in raising it to give a toast he is apt to fall into a very absurd gesture. He lifts the hand containing the glass without considering that fluids are not solid bodies ; and after he, in any event, would have spilled the contents by this movement, he enacts the pantomime of drinking. Nothing can be more absurd than this. One has only to take a really full glass in hand and note how different will be the gesture. The glass is certainly raised at the toast, not with a jerk, however, but with a gentle arm-movement.

Many commit just as great an error when sitting before a full pitcher or cup from which they must drink for a long time ; they make at the first or second draught, a movement indicating that the liquid is all gone, and after this pretend to drink from the already empty vessel. This must be carefully avoided.

If the actor has to drink continuously from a glass or mug, without power to refill it, he must reckon exactly how he may represent the gradual exhaustion of the vessel. This must also be observed in pouring wine from a bottle or pitcher. The second pouring usually gives the spectator an idea that the vessel is empty, and yet we see the actor go on making the motion of pouring from the empty bottle.

GESTURE.

Neither must the drinker, as a man of the world, bend his head down to the cup; he must carry it to his mouth. If the drinking is characteristic, if it is to represent an extraordinary thirst, a sort of eagerness, the head must be bent toward the cup more or less according to the degree of thirst, or the lower or higher rank of the person.

Trivial as these faults are, they are, nevertheless, faults, and the actor must not suppose that they escape the close observer. They excite a smile, the smile leads to a laugh, which called forth in the wrong place will spoil everything.

2. *The Holding of a Cup of Coffee or Tea.*

If a cup is to be finely held, the spoon must not be placed in the saucer, but must remain in the cup. The saucer is held with the left hand, the cup with the right (Fig. LXII.) and is carried

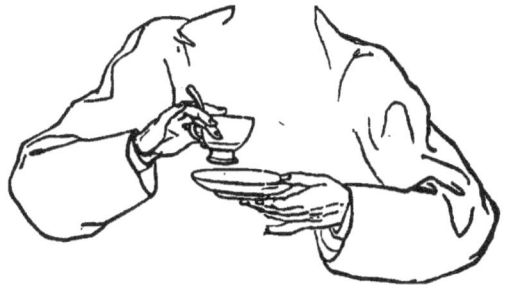

FIG. LXII.

to the mouth without bending the head toward the cup, and replaced the same way in the saucer. To take sugar with the fingers is always "bad form."

3. *Patomimic Reading and Letter Writing.*

Both, as a general thing, occur upon the stage in so remarkably short a time that it is impossible for the spectator to believe in the truth of what he sees.

Reading.— Every letter has a superscription. Let the letter contain what it will ; it may set the reader into ever so much excitement (sorrow, joy, pain, etc.,) he usually reads its superscription calmly, if it does not of itself prophesy misfortune, or the reader does not already know that misfortune awaits him. Here a pause, be it ever so short, is necessary ; then begins the pantomime of reading the letter. Whether it is long or short, the effect must in this way be visible to the spectators. The actor has exactly to indicate the preface, the continuation and at last the culmination of the letter, if ever so short, before he passes over to its effect in the pantomime. But as we see constantly, especially in opera letter reading, the opening and the patomime of the climax are one, and the reading takes place with a rapidity that in real life would not suffice for reading the simplest superscription. The tragic situation thus becomes comic.

Writing.— In just such an unnatural way writing takes place upon the stage. If the actor has not as much time as the writing of the letter really demands, he must strictly hold to the required stage time if he would not destroy all illusions. But most letters are written in as short a time as the mere signature of the writer would demand. We seldom see the letter dried in pantomime by sand or blotting paper, and the audience have the involuntary feeling that its receiver receives a blotted, illegible letter, which is against the laws of good breeding. If the actor has no blotting paper upon his desk, he must go through the patomime of using sand. But he must not forget to shake off the sand, for it is as bad form to send a letter full of sand as a blotted one.

"One thing I implore, no more sand upon the little notes you write to me ! To-day I quickly passed it to my lips, and my teeth grated." (Werther to Lotte.)

Here Goethe is only in jest, but it is really not nice to show sand upon a letter, nor quite respectful to a superior. It is better to use blotting paper which should be upon every writing-table. If neither is at hand, the actor must make a slight movement through the air, to hint at least at drying ; and a hint suffices on the stage.

4. *Turning the Leaves of a Book.*

Many in real life have the habit of moistening the finger at the mouth in turning a leaf, and carry this habit to the stage. The reason of this is a fear that two leaves may be turned instead of one. It is a habit wounding to fine sensibilities, and upon the stage, where there should always be the semblance of good society, it is more offensive than in real life. The leaf to be turned must not be seized at the very moment of turning, but some time in advance thereof, and in the following manner : Lay the thumb lightly on the leaf to be turned, and at its upper edge sever it lightly from the others with the index and middle fingers.

5. *Use of a Pencil.*

It is just as ill-mannered to moisten the pencil at the mouth, from time to time. If the pencil is good it will do its work unmoistened ; if bad, moistening is of no use, for it must follow every word, and how would such writing look ?

These are slight faults, but if one aspires to high and noble things, he must avoid them.

PRACTICAL EXERCISES FOR PUPILS.

If the pupil has mastered the first three parts of our book, the preparatory steps demanded by our system are nearly ended. His next step must be a practical application of what he has learned,—by gestures and movements without words.

A few examples will illustrate our demand. We take these from Fred. Ludwig Schmidt's, "Aphorisms," a book to be warmly commended to every disciple of art, that is to say, after he has mastered perfectly the three above mentioned parts of our book. Otherwise the following and all similar demands made upon the pupil will be useless work to both pupil and teacher. These trials are :

1. A simple entrance, a walking forward, the handing of a let-

ter, the reception of a hint to leave, turning with respect to one or several persons in the room.

2. The pupil tries an entrance in his own character. He imagines that he enters a hall containing a brilliant assemblage. How many grades of movement, how many of bearing are supposable here? Decorous walking forward in itself; bowing in general, then in particular to the mistress and master of the house, to a distinguished guest, to an acquaintance, a relative; each situation demands ever so subtle, yet a different movement. If one will pursue this business still further, he may imagine some event; it may be to pick up a fallen card and hand it over properly (see Part Third); to bring a chair to a lady, or to conduct her with the required gallantry to a sofa. Many such cases are at hand and can be utilized by the pupil.

3. The pupil walks slowly in at the door, lingers here in an uneasy attitude, strides forward with interrupted steps, then falls slowly down on the left knee (if the object of his homage is at his right). He now imagines her flying to his left; he rises anxiously, follows with quickened steps, and ventures here a sudden fall, using the right knee, lingers entreating, then rises quickly, makes a movement to go, tarries, glances back and now hastens from the stage. In this practice a change in step or gait is to be accurately observed. The teacher allows a pause at every change of attitude, and arranges the proper carriage of the whole body with constant care to its always appearing half turned toward the parquet.

4. The pupil paces the stage in a passionate mood, strides over it in all directions, makes a longer or shorter pause at each, throws himself exhausted upon a sofa, springs up, hastens in towering passion to the door, feigns meeting a horrible object here and swoons.

Here would be the whole gamut from the first calm step to the wild plunge. This it is which is learned from no dancing master;— to which only a skilled artist can lead the way, by whom the practice only briefly hinted at here may be indefinitely extended.

The next practice in mimic representation is confined to certain passions which the teacher gives at will, mounting from easy to difficult, expanding them in all directions ; proving whether the pupil can put to practical use all he has learned or must be helped here and there, and where.

If the teacher is convinced that the pupil satisfies these demands, and the latter has brought his voice and speaking apparatus to the same degree of cultivation as his body, then he may proceed to the third step of culture in which words are united to gesture ; to dramatic representation, passing on systematically from the easy to the difficult.

If the pupil is educated by another than this rational method, as has mostly been the case hitherto, his future depends upon accident ; he will waste his best years in a search for laws which have nothing to do with the fundamental principles of the actor's art. In coming and going, in twisting and turning, in the carriage and movements of the arms, we still recognize the beginner even after years. Yes, he not seldom betrays it in minor things, by falling into mannerisms,— and magnificent talents are in this way lost for dramatic art.

PART FOURTH.

THE ART OF DANCING.

CHAPTER I.

THE ART OF DANCING.

Dancing is usually divided into two sorts :
1. The Society and National Dance.
2. The Theatrical Dance.

Although almost every country has a peculiar kind of society dance, they are all alike in that two or more persons take certain prescribed steps, more or less complicated, to musical *tempo*, and repeated *ad libitum*.

We find the dance in the most ancient times, but naturally in a simple form. In the middle ages it fell into disuse, not reviving until the seventeenth century, and then in Italy, from whence it went to France and there attained the high perfection it enjoys to-day.

1. Carriage of the Body.

The Upper Body.—It is important in ordinary life that the body and its limbs should appear only in plastic attitudes, but this is especially requisite in the art of dancing. A carriage erect but without stiffness, an easy, unembarrassed bearing of the arms, a pleasing and agreeable position of the hands and fingers are indispensably essential. We attain these by expanding the chest, throwing back the shoulders, and letting the head set lightly and easily upon the shoulders.

The character dance certainly demands various positions of the body ; but elasticity, grace and decorum are main conditions which even in the rudest national dance must not be wanting. If one pretends to the name of artist, these must be strictly observed.

Legs and Feet.—The main rule is that from the hips to the thigh and knee, the upper legs must be turned sharply outward, whereby the lower legs and toes are forced into the same position

2. *Fundamental Positions and Movements.*

There are five positions of the feet and three of the arms, the third of which is of a twofold sort; and four fundamental movements, viz.: Two knee-movements, bending and extending (every dance-movement begins with bending and ends with extending); and two movements of foot-bending, including the toes — up and down tension. From these fundamental attitudes and movements arise the fundamental steps.

As seven notes form the foundation of the art of music, so seven steps form the basis of the present art of dancing; and new and complicated steps arise only from the quicker or slower transition from the one to the other, the blending of two or more steps, and the more or less frequent repetition of the one step or the other.

3. *The Position of the Feet.*

First Position.—Both heels together, the toes as far apart as possible. (Fig. LXIII.) Every other position of the toes, so

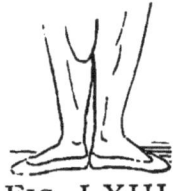

FIG. LXIII.

that the heels only remain closed, is also called the first position.

Second Position.— The right or left foot in a straight line sideward. (Fig. LXIV.)

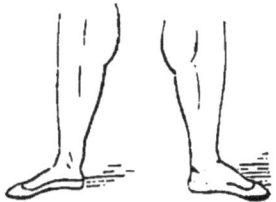

Fig. LXIV.

Third Position.— The heel of one foot stands by the inward middle of the other. (Fig. LXV.)

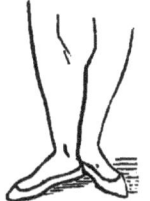

FIG. LXV.

Fourth Position.— Like the third, with the difference that the feet are separated. (Fig. LXVI.)

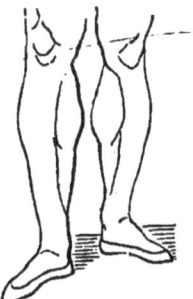

FIG. LXVI.

Fifth Position.— The toes sharply turned outward, press one of them against the heel of the other foot. (Fig. LXVII.)

While the first four positions are met with at every moment of daily life, the fifth position is found in the dancing art only, where it passes as a proof of artistic dexterity.

The positions are also divided into closed and open. The closed are the *first*, *third* and *fifth*; the open, the *second* and *fourth*. The removal of the foot into the open position is made according to the size of the body, and will be right if the knees remain tense and the bodily carriage is natural.

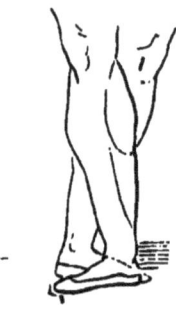

Fig. LXVII.

From the four fundamental movements — bending, extending tension up and down — arise eight main movements. These render possible every action of the foot out of the fundamental position, remaining in one place or taking various directions, and are named as follows:—

(*a*) The right; a direct line forward and backward.

(*b*) Open; spread to the sideward, right and left.

(*c*) Round; circular formed.

(*d*) Tortuous; in serpentine windings.

(*e*) Slippery; slipping, gliding, grazing.

(*f*) Leaping and falling back; hopping or springing upward, and, in consequence, again falling back or down.

(*g*) *Tourné;* turning with swinging motion.

(*h*) *Battu;* beating in the widest sense; that is, beating outward, inward, toward, or together.

4. The Position of the Arms.

First position.— The arms hang unrestrained and lightly at the side. (Fig. LXVII. *a,— d, e;* also Fig. XXXII.; *a, c* and Figs. X. and X. *a,* 1.)

DANCING. 143

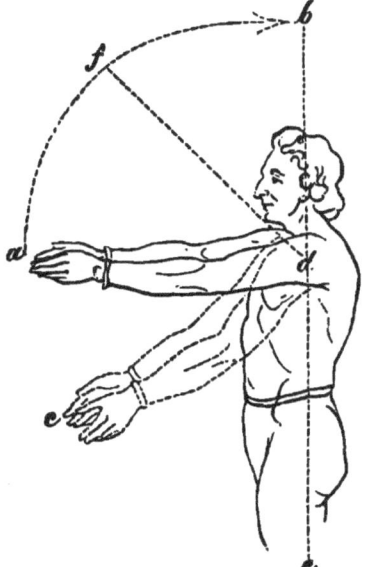

Fig. LXVII. *a*.

Second Position.— Both arms swing horizontally at the side, the thumbs upward. (Fig XXVII., 4, 4.)

Third Position (*a*).— The arms swing horizontally forward a shoulder's breadth from each other. (Fig. LXVII. *a*,— *d*, *a*.)

Third Position (*b*).— The arms are equally removed from each other, perpendicularly at the sides of the head. (Fig. LXVII. *a*,— *d*, *b*.)

This position, as well as the transition from the second position (also from the third position *a*) to the third position (*b*) indicates, in pantomime, only exaltation (high passion), and finds no application in society dances.

We found in Æsthetic Gymnastics the application of the positions of the arms; here it may only be remarked that in their execution an avoidance of all angles and an easy, agreeable, rounded form are the main conditions.

5. *Exercises Preliminary to the Dance.*

If the pupil has thoroughly pursued the course of gymnastics laid down in Part Second, in learning to dance he will only need to add artistic forms and to reduce to formulas what he has already learned.

The most excellent practices are :—

For the Arms.— Facility in the carriage and movement of the arms, avoiding everything forced and exaggerated and all angles and sprawling, acquiring the ability to pass from one position to another in rounded and swaying lines (Hogarthian line of beauty), is called in dancing the *port de bras.*

We divide the *port de bras* into the lower (Fig. XXVII., 4, 4) and into the higher (Fig. XXVII., 3.) Under the first head we include all movements that take place below, or horizontal to, the shoulders, either before, or sideward to, them; under the second head, movements above the shoulders, forward or sideward. Hence the first, second and third position (*a*) form the lower *port de bras*, while the third position (*b*) alone forms the higher. In society dances only the lower *port de bras* appears; the higher only in artistic and national dances. In artistic dances it is to be especially cultivated, inasmuch as the greatest readiness in the use of the legs loses its effect through a bad *port de bras*.

The practice for the lower *port de bras* is : Fifth position of the feet, first position of the arms. After lifting the arms in the way prescribed in Part II. to the region of the shoulders, they are allowed to fall lightly and gracefully into the second position. (Fig. XXVII., 4, 4.) They remain a while in this position, then make a change of feet (see elementary dancing step), and pass slowly back to the first position. (Fig. XXVII., 4, 5, 6, and 1.) Then the same is done with each arm.

The gymnastic practice of Part II. leads us to the high *port de bras*. In order to acquire the requisite skill and *roundness* for this, one holds the arms extended over the head (Fig. XXVII., 3) for some time, then marches, according to the rules for walking, several times to and fro, and then resumes the normal position.

We here call attention once more to the remarks in Physical Gymnastics (Part II.), exactly prescribing the carriage of the arms and hands. An easy carriage of the hands is here indispensable.

The *port de bras* is also practiced in every one of the five fundamental positions, and makes with the third and fifth a *changement de pieds*.

We again repeat that the pupil cannot often enough practice the *port de bras*, for this forms the basis of all arm movements. (Fig. XXXII.)

For the Feet. — In Physical Gymnastics we learned the upward and downward tension of the foot-joint, and there is nothing further to add save that it must here be still more light and pleasing.

Bending and stretching the knee is practiced in all the five fundamental positions, and always in such a way that the outward turned knee forms a direct line with the toes. In passing from bending to stretching the heel is lifted somewhat to throw the centre of gravity wholly upon the toes. The exercises given in Part II. have prepared us to execute this bending and stretching with ease.

Under the term *battements* we understand the striking movements of the legs; two wholly opposite movements making one *battement*. They are divided into small and great. To practice them correctly, one grasps some fixed object with one hand (perhaps it is a bar at the height of the hips, and made fast to the wall, or the back of a chair, with the seat turned to the wall), and performs the practice with the opposite leg, until he can carry it through standing without support.

Petits Battements. — Position: Second position, one foot suspended, with the toes indicating the second position, the other firmly sustaining the body. At a two *tempo*, the suspended foot with bended knee strikes into the fifth position before or behind the standing foot, and by quick, energetic stretching, back into the second position, still suspended. The heel must be strongly pressed forward, the knee outward.

Grands Battements. — While the small *battements* are executed only sideward, the great ones are in a threefold way: forward, backward, and sideward.

Forward *battement:* The foot standing forward in the fifth position, strikes energetically forward, with stretched (tense) knee as high as possible, and immediately falls back into the fifth position. It may be remarked here that, in raising the foot, the toe leaves the floor last; in setting it down, touches the floor first.

Backward: Like the forward, only that the movement is made with the hindmost foot. This *battement*, on account of the structure of the body, can be executed only in a limited way. Still, by early practice, a considerable height may be reached.

Sideward: Like the forward, with the arms held in the second position.

Ronds de jambe are of two sorts — inner and outer. The suspended foot held in the second position, passes the standing foot in a circle, from back to front, or vice versa, so that at the outer part of the circle the toes alone lightly touch the floor, while the heel also does the same near the standing foot. Of course, this can happen only through the active aid of the foot-joint.

For the Upper Body. — We have treated of *turning upon the hips* in Part II. as "Turning the Torso." We only add here that this must be practiced in all five positions. In the first and fourth positions of the feet, the hands are planted at the hips; in the second, third, and fifth, the arms assume the second position (Fig. XXVII., 4, 4).

For the Whole Body. — The easy and graceful transition of the centre of gravity from one foot to the other, is called *disengaging*. It appears especially in the two open positions, the second and fourth. It is to be remarked that if a disengagement takes place in the fourth position, in which case the centre of gravity will be transferred from the backward to the forward foot, the former touches the floor only with the great toe, and as the centre of gravity passes from the forward to the backward foot, the latter (the forward foot) touches the floor with the little toe.

In our walking backward, in Part I., we have prepared for this movement, and have only to observe greater exactness in respect to the toes.

6. Single Movements of the Feet Through Which the Dancing Steps are Rendered Possible.

The Walking Step. — If, in passing forward, backward or sideways, one transfers the centre of gravity from one foot to the other, he has taken a step. The soldier's "halt" is, therefore, only a downward drawing or "fastening" of the foot after the last step.

The walking step of the dance is executed in the following manner: After a slight bending of both knees, one foot rises, the heel first, and passes into the fourth or second position, resting upon the toes; and while the centre of gravity is transferred to this, the heel lightly falls downward. This is the step already referred to in walking upon the stage.

Besides this simple, common step, there are five others which form the transition to the dance. Klemm names them as follows:

Les pas balancés, the swaying, rocking step forward and backward.

Les pas sur les pointes, upon the toes forward and backward.

Les pas élevés, the lifted, skipping step.

Les pas sautés, springing forward and backward.

Les pas soutenus, slipping, continuous steps forward and backward.

7. Elementary Dancing Steps.

The changement de pieds (changing of the feet) is a spring in one *tempo*, as a rule, into the third or fifth position. Its execution in the third and fifth positions happens in the following way : a slight bending of both knees, then a swing of both feet more or less high, and a passing to the original position, with a change of feet.

If, through much practice, the foot-joint and the toes have attained great elasticity, this change of feet may take place without lifting the toes from the floor.

The *assemblé* is the uniting of both feet from an open to a closed position in one *tempo*. Its main condition is that the standing foot should always, after bending the knees, swing upward and be set upon the floor directly with the other.

The *glissade* is a dancing step composed of two others, the second of which receives the most accent, and the first, as a rule, begins in advance of a bar.

The *glissade* is, for the most part, executed from right to left, but it can, like all elementary steps, be executed in all directions. Its manner of execution is as follows :

Both knees being bent slightly, the right foot sways over into the second position, as if it would step over some object, rests there upon the toes, and draws the other foot after it into the fifth position, while it (the right) lets itself down on its heel. The left foot that slips after, can only be brought before or behind the right one, into the fifth position.

The *jeté*, a step similar to running and springing, is the upward swing of one foot of a closed position, while the other, passing into one of the two open positions, falls back directly into the closed position in one *tempo*.

(Let it be remarked here, that in all practice in the third, fourth and fifth positions, the right foot is always supposed to be forward.)

Execution : Fifth position, during the slight bending of both knees, the left foot, throwing itself sideways and swaying into the second position, falls immediately into the fifth position before the right foot, while this one, swaying behind the left foot, remains in the fifth position.

The *chassé* is the chasing of the one foot of an open position by the other into an again open position in two *tempi*, and is thus executed: Fourth position, centre of gravity upon the left foot. While the centre of gravity is lightly and gracefully transferred to the right foot, and the left, after a slight bending and consequent light up-swinging of both feet, is thrown back into the third position, the right foot again passes forward into the fourth position. The setting downward of the left foot happens at the first, the setting forward of the right foot at the second *tempo*. In several successive *chassés*, an exchange of the feet naturally takes place.

In the backward *chassé*, if the centre of gravity is on the forward foot, it will pass over to the hindmost one, and chase this from its place, which then becomes the foremost. In the sideward *chassé*, the foot to be *chasséd* must stand in the second position.

The *temps de cuisse* is a movement in two *tempi* from a closed position into an up-swinging one, with the two feet falling back upon one foot, so that the one foot is held upward in the second or fourth position, and then falls forward or backward into the fifth.

Execution: Second position, the centre of gravity upon the right foot, the left suspended and tense. While the right foot bends slightly, the left, with the powerful aid of the upper leg, strikes forcibly backward with the toes into the second position (upon the floor); but in a moment rises again and passes, while the right, in a slight up-swinging and with a short step, springs to the right, into the third or fifth position, before or behind the right foot. A sideward *temps de cuisse* must always be preceded by a *jeté*, and is then called *zephyr step* — (*pas de zéphire*).

The *pas de bourrée* is a step with three movements. Execution: Fifth position, the right foot rises, with a slight bending of the left knee, suspended in the second position, falls backward into the fifth position, raising itself with stretched knees and upon both toes, then drawing the left into the second, and the right into the fifth position.

All these steps may be executed forward, backward, sideward, in turning, walking, slipping and springing, simple, double, three, four, and manifold *tempo* (as often as possible), and form, in this way, the art of dancing.

8. *Composite Independent Steps.*

Besides these seven fundamental steps, a knowledge of two others is necessary — the *echappé* and the *pas de basque*.

The *echappé* is really a fundamental step, but as several *echappés* in succession may be formed only if an *assemblé* takes place between any two, we call it a composite independent, but not a fundamental step. It is the simultaneous up-swinging of both feet out of a closed position into an open, upon one *tempo*. Its execution is as follows: For example, Fifth position, after the preparatory bending (bowing), both feet swing upward from the floor, and fall into an open position.

The *pas de basque* is composed of two steps and a closing one, to be executed in two *tempi*. It can be executed in all directions. The forward execution requires the fifth position. In advance of the bar, bending of both knees, and throwing the right foot into the fourth position; hereupon the left foot passes lightly and gracefully, both knees again being stretched, past the right foot into the fourth position, assumes the centre of gravity, and immediately the right foot closes into the fifth position, and a *pas de basque* is ended. If several succeed one another, the left foot must naturally be placed into the fourth position.

Backward. — The same steps, only in the opposite movement. The left foot, standing behind in the fifth position, begins, while it falls into the fourth position; the right goes backward past this into the fourth position, and the left immediately closes into the fifth position before the right foot.

All other steps occurring in the art of dancing are variations of these seven fundamental steps. To explain them is foreign to the purpose of our book.

9. *The Minuet as a School for Compliments.*

The minuet is a dance of two persons, moving in slow, dignified, walking steps. It is of French origin, was carried to the highest perfection under Louis XIV. and Louis XV., and has now entirely vanished from the array of society dances.

In the last century, a knowledge of the minuet was indispensable for every cultivated person. All movements of the body, especially those of the feet and arms, required at court or in polite assemblies, consisted in those of the minuet. Every ceremonial bow must be the "reverence" of the minuet. It was, therefore, the school of fine manners.

It cannot be denied that the product of this school was an exaggerated etiquette — even a painful stiffness — which, thank heaven! has vanished from the circles of the present day; but, on the other hand, it cannot be denied that, for this very reason, outward decorum has suffered.

If we would learn the manners of good society in modern days, we can do no better than to learn them through the minuet; for this still forms, and always will, the basis of all *tournure*.

To describe the minuet in its infinite, various forms, would be against the purpose of our book. We have here to treat only of a part of it, that which preceded every minuet, the "reverence."

10. *Compliment — Reverence.*

A salutation without words, that is, a mere more or less profound bowing of the body, is called a *compliment*. The second signification of the compliment, to say a polite or pleasant thing to some one, does not come within our province.

We make this distinction of dates: The compliment (salutation) of ancient times, the compliment of the middle ages, the compliment of the seventeenth and eighteenth centuries, and the modern compliment.

The Compliment of Ancient Times. — This had two degrees : (1) the friendly greeting ; and (2) the ceremonial (polite) greeting, the sign of high respect and reverence. The first degree was shown by a slight step forward, the head being somewhat bowed, and the inclination of the body but slight. Here one arm, with the palm of the hand upward, approaches the object, while the other remains passive, or is placed in protestation (of regard) upon the breast. This was the friendly greeting of ancient times, as represented in *bas reliefs*. If this were transformed into a polite (or ceremonial) greeting, the head of the woman bowed more deeply than that of the man ; the greeting arm was more outstretched, and the knees bowed more deeply. With a man the head remained more erect, the neck more stretched forward, the glance fixed upon the highly respected object, and the knee of the backward leg bent more than the forward one.

The Mediæval Compliment. — This consisted in bending the knee, and had three degrees :

(1) An entire falling upon the knees, as the highest degree of reverence and salutation (Fig. LXVIII.). (2) The bending of the one knee (Fig. LXIX.). It is thus executed : One walks forward sideways, with one foot or the other (here in Fig. LXIX., with the right), assuming the centre of gravity, and while with the other foot (here in Fig. LXIX., the left) he goes in a line slightly bent outward to the designated point, the inclination takes place. (3) The mere bowing of the body with one foot set back upon the toes (as in Fig. LXX.).

In all three gradations, we find the same movement of the right hand, the laying it upon the breast ; but in an entire falling upon the knees in passion, the right hand is outstretched to the one saluted, in token of the fullest reverence and veneration, as the sign of unconditional submission. (See Fig. LXVIII.) Still this is not indispensably necessary ; the hand may lie as in

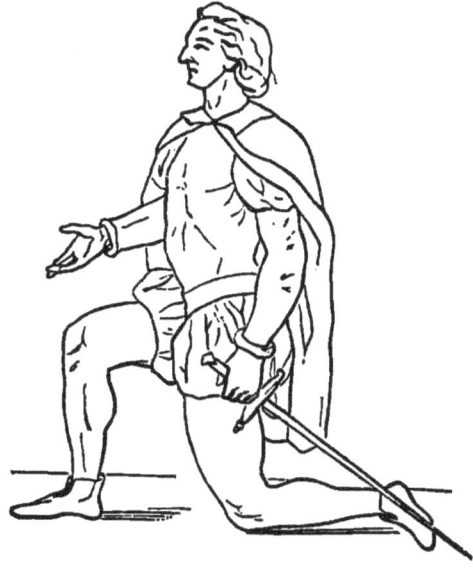

FIG. LXVIII.

Fig. LXIX. For position of fingers of the right hand, we refer to Fig. XXXIX.

The lady has just the same to do. A modern compliment would be entirely wrong.

After this brief description of the mediæval compliment, it must occur to every one how senseless it is, when we see upon the stage, a mailed knight, a true mediæval figure, pay the modern compliment, or a castle lady execute the reverence of the *rococo* age. Thus, for instance, in "Don Carlos," and similar pieces, no compliment must be made, but falling on the knees, according to the necessary gradations.

The Compliment of the Seventeenth and Eighteenth Centuries (in France, the Regime of Louis XIV., XV., and XVI.). — In this age we find the compliment in its highest cultivation; it preceded every minuet, and had two gradations :

(1) The Great Reverence.

154 ÆSTHETIC PHYSICAL CULTURE.

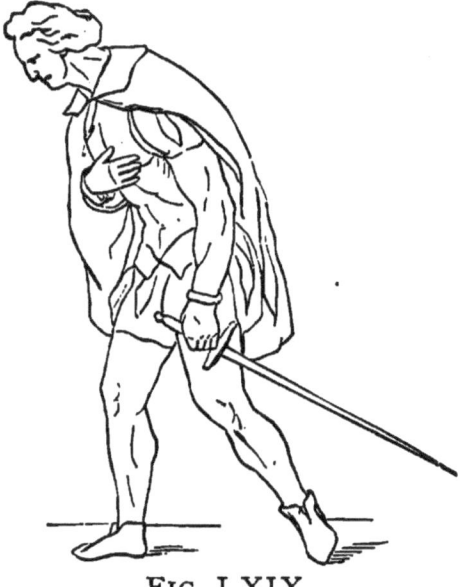

FIG. LXIX.

(2) The Little Reverence.

The execution (strictly in time, even if no music was at hand) demanded twice as much time in the first degree as the last.

The Great Reverence for Gentlemen. — The right or left foot (the right in the minuet) passes, after a slight bending of both knees in advance of the bar, into the second position, taking up the centre of gravity. The other (in the minuet, the left) foot will be slowly drawn over into the first position, while the body bends forward. During these times, the right hand of the gentleman (if it does not hold the hand of the lady) grasps the hat resting under the left arm, and passes into the movement of salutation, to the right side. (Fig. LXXI.) Now follows the return of the body to its erect posture, while the left foot, after a slight bending and stretching of both knees, takes a step backward into the fourth position upon the toes, and then upon the heel, assuming the centre of gravity, and the right hand has car-

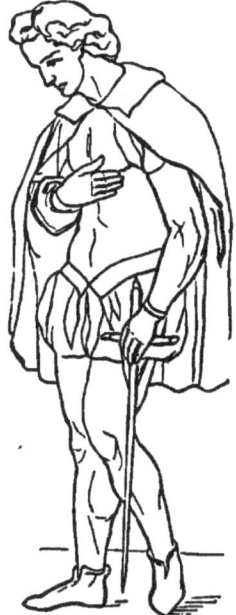

FIG. LXX.

ried the hat back, under the left arm, to its former place. (Fig. LXXII.) Then the foot, standing forward in the fourth position, is again drawn over into the third position, and the right hand is again brought to the right side.

In the minuet, if the gentleman holds the lady with his right hand, the hat naturally remains quietly under the left arm.

The bowing itself must take place in the following way: The head inclines forward and draws the shoulders slowly after it; but if the bowing takes place from the waist, the upper and lower body forms an obtuse angle, which must not happen, as it is always the sign of awkwardness. In again rising erect, head and glance give the impulse.

Before princes, and in the presence of persons of high rank,

156   ÆSTHETIC PHYSICAL CULTURE.

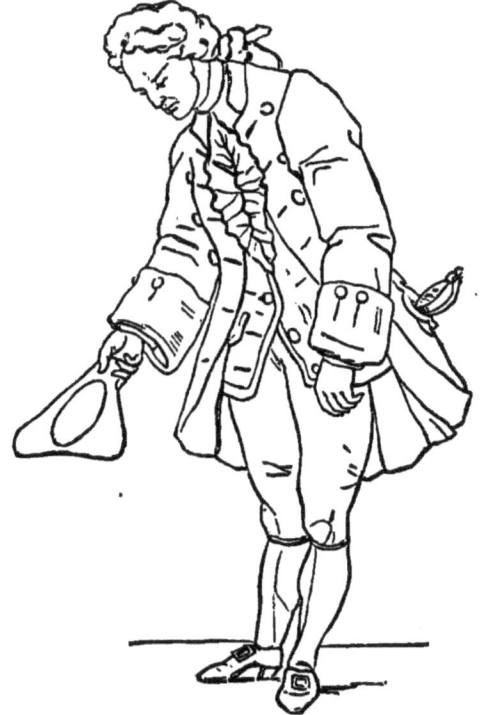

Fig. LXXI.

the bow is more significant; still it must not be supposed that greater reverence is expressed by too profound bowing. A slower inclination, with a slower drawing on of the foot, and a like slowness in resuming the erect attitude, is the sign of great respect.

The Great Reverence for Ladies. — This, always begun in the third position, is a deep bending of both knees, with erect upper body (the characteristic of this compliment), a stepping backward upon one foot, and resuming the erect attitude.

It is thus executed: After a slight bending and stretching of both knees, the right or left foot (in the minuet, the right) passes

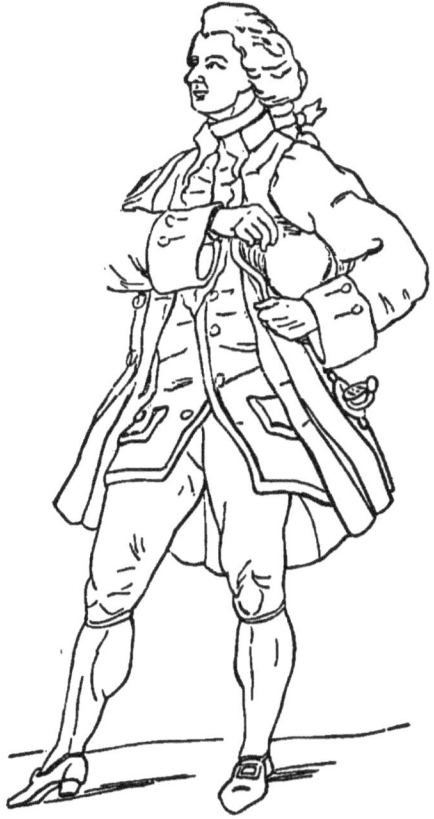

Fig. LXXII.

into the second position, assuming the centre of gravity, while the other is drawn over into the third position ; then deep bending, the upper body held erect (Fig. LXXIII.); then stepping back upon one or the other foot (in the first reverence of the minuet upon the right), during which a slight inclination of the body takes place, and which already happens in rising (Fig. LXXIII., *a*) and a drawing on of the forward standing foot into the third position. (Fig. LXXIII., *b*.)

158   ÆSTHETIC PHYSICAL CULTURE.

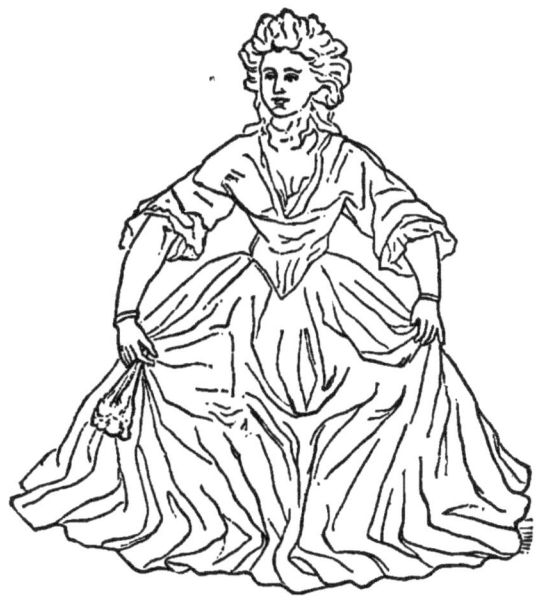

FIG. LXXIII.

The index finger and thumb hold, meantime, both sides of the dress, drawing it gracefully away from the body; in the minuet, only the right hand holds the dress, while the left is reached to the gentleman. The manner of holding the fan is shown in Fig. LXXIII.

The deeper and slower the bowing, the greater the respect.

To make the ladies' reverence in such a way that, in bowing, the upper part of the body bends forward, is especially false.

If the lady stands in an open position, she must first step into a closed (the third), and then the reverence begins.

The Little Reverence for Gentlemen. — The right or left foot (without a previous bending and extension of both knees) passes into the second position upon the toes, then upon the heel, assuming the centre of gravity. Then the other foot will be drawn into the first position, while the bowing itself takes place.

DANCING.   159

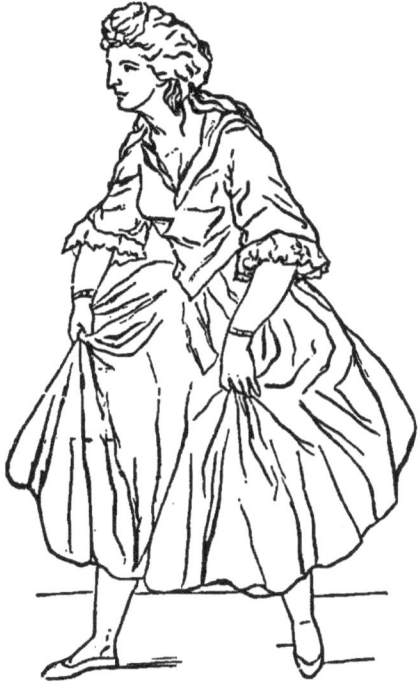

FIG. LXXIII. *a*.

The Little Reverence for Ladies. — Like the great reverence, only without the slight bending and stretching of both knees, and the consequent steps sideward, beginning in the closed position, with the deep bow, the upper body being held erect, and stepping back on one foot or the other, etc.

The Little Reverence (*sideway*). — For gentlemen, this is like the great reverence, only with the difference that, at the outset, the foot to be set into the second position is here (while turning the body) placed sideward-backward upon the toes, then upon the heel, assuming the centre of gravity; by drawing on the other foot and bowing, the compliment is executed.

160   ÆSTHETIC PHYSICAL CULTURE.

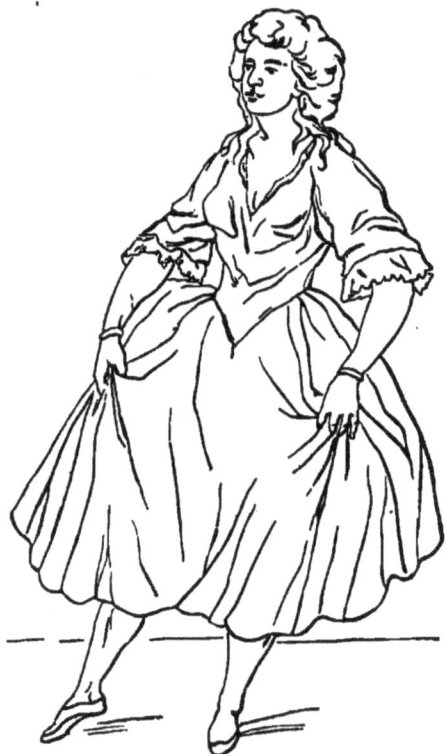

FIG. LXXIII. b.

If ladies have to make the little reverence sideward, the preparatory step must likewise be taken sideward-backward, with a turning of the body; thus the other foot will be drawn into the closed position, and the low bowing, etc., follow.

These are the main compliments before *one* person. If several are to be greeted, little changes enter, which, with gentlemen and ladies, are as follows:

Reverence before Several Persons Standing in a Half-Circle.—
The simple reverence: The drawing forward of the foot and bowing in gentlemen, the bending and setting back of the foot in

ladies, must take place more slowly, while glance and body, which, at the beginning of the reverence, are fixed upon the first person, while the bow takes place, turn slowly and in a dignified manner to the last person of the semi-circle, where the bow ends, the upright position being resumed by a slight turning back to the middle of the semi-circle.

In glancing from left to right in the semi-circle, with gentlemen, the left foot must step into the second position, and the right be drawn after it; with ladies, after bowing, the right foot must be set back. In glancing from the right to the left, the order is reversed.

The double reverence: If two compliments are to be made in succession (the one to the right, the other to the left), a turning of the body upon the ball of the foot must take place between those to whom the bower turns. Naturally with gentlemen, at the beginning of the second compliment, the foot nearest the side takes the second position, and with ladies, if, at the first compliment, the left foot had stepped back, now, after bowing, the right foot steps back.

The Little Reverence upon Arrival. — This is like the main compliment. The gentleman has only to observe that the last step in arrival is somewhat slower and sideway-forward, instead of forward; it will serve as the first step of the beginning compliment, upon which the drawing forward of the other foot, and the bow itself, follow.

The lady walks to the point where she has to make the compliment in the third position, and immediately begins the compliment with a bow. If the great reverence is to be made upon arrival, the lady and gentleman pass in a direct line to the place where it is to be executed.

The Little Reverence, at Departure, for Gentlemen. — The compliment itself is like the main compliment, only it is preceded by one step backward, while the second, instead of following in a direct line, passes sideward-backward into the fourth position;

now, as in the main compliment, follow the drawing on of the other foot, and the bowing. The third step now succeeding may (if the space is large enough) take place upon a direct line backward, without turning. If this is not the case, it is made with turning toward the exit; not a full, but a half turn, and now follow, as space allows, one or two steps to complete the turn.

The great reverence is likewise preceded by one step backward, followed by a drawing on of the foremost foot into the first position, and at once begin the slight "bending and stretching" of both knees, the sideward stepping into the second position, etc.

The Little Reverence, at Departure, for Ladies. — This likewise demands a step backward, and a drawing of the foremost foot again into the third position. Now begins the deep bending without stepping sideward, then stepping back, etc. The great reverence is made with stepping sideward.

After the compliment, there is likewise one step backward, which is the continuation of the drawing back of the foremost foot, which has at once passed by the standing foot back into the fourth position. The turning is as with gentlemen.

These are the compliments which all, more or less, are to be executed like the main compliment. Whether the great or little reverence is to be made, depends always upon the person to be saluted as well as upon the situation. Exalted persons, grave situations, demand the great reverence.

Reverence at Meeting in Walking. — For Gentlemen and Ladies. — Before one person: The head and upper body are slightly turned toward the person to be greeted, while the walk becomes slower, but does not cease; while the foot upon this side slides a little out of the direct line of walking until one is past. In the salons of the *rococo* time the waving of the hand with the hat, as described in the minuet, followed, and removing the hat when in the open air.

Before a prince, one steps aside, halts, then "makes front," and salutes him.

Before several persons : If one walks past a row of persons, sitting or standing, the same rule will be observed ; only with the difference that both feet pass into the *glissé* step, until he is past.

Passing between two rows : If one passes between two rows, he must, alternately, with the right and left foot, execute the *glissé* step, until he is past, and at each change of foot turn to those he would salute, as before described.

Reverence in Sitting. — For Gentlemen and Ladies. — This appears only in the society of friends and familiar acquaintances, or if, in sitting at table, something is reached to us, and we cannot rise ; also, when princes or persons of high standing greet those of lower rank.

It consists of a mere bending of the upper part of the body and head, with a corresponding glance, the bow being more or less deep, according to circumstances, but not a mere hasty nod, which is allowed only by the highest degree of familiarity.

Whether the actor has to make the great or little reverence, must be left to his own decision.

The Modern Compliment. — Our time has certainly much simplified the compliment, but if we lay any claim to culture, we must not go so far as to let a mere drawing together of the heels, with a slight, superficial bow, pass as a compliment. Our compliment, both with ladies and gentlemen, is the little reverence of the *rococo* age ; still with a slight variation. The lady no longer takes hold of her dress to draw it aside somewhat ; she no longer bows so profoundly, or with an erect position of the upper part of the body, but with simultaneous bending ; this principally distinguishes it from the *rococo* compliment.

The gentleman lets his hands hang easily at the side, according to the mere law of gravity. (Fig. LXXIV.)

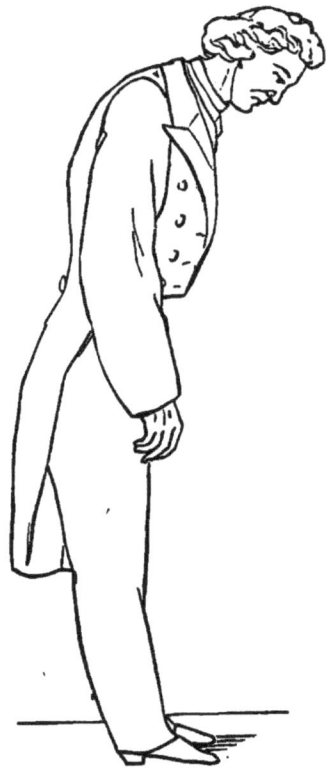

Fig. LXXIV.

This is our main compliment of modern times. In all other respects, we observe to-day the precepts of the *rococo* age.

We must not neglect to warn against that jerky, backward movement, which robs the compliment of all significance. In the age of the minuet, such a warning would have been superfluous, as every cultured person had the time in feeling, if not in music, and paid heed to it.

A slight pause must ensue between the bowing and the rising erect again.

To execute the modern gentleman's compliment, without having first stepped with one or the other foot into the second position, that is, in the first or third, is altogether wrong.

If the gentleman already stands in the second position, he passes with one foot into the fourth position (using this advance as the preparatory position — for the compliment must not be made without preparation ; and if the space is limited, the step must be made shorter), and then draws the other foot into the first position.

If the lady stands in the second or fourth position, she draws one foot past the other into a closed (third) position, and now makes the bending, etc.

If the gentleman stands in the fourth position, he passes with the foremost foot into the second (for the sake of preparation), and draws the other into the first position.

The various gestures with which a silent bowing can be accompanied, belong to special mimic art, with a description of which our book has nothing to do. Here let it only be remarked, that those hand-movements so constantly recurring especially upon the stage, as if one would reach something to the person greeted, are altogether inadmissible, and, at most, may be used by persons of high station, when they would show a sort of friendly condescension or good will to those of lower station ; or if a princess greets those around her, in which case, she makes the accompanying gesture with her fan, or merely with the hand. It is also allowed in familiarity, but never in a person of lower toward one of a higher rank.

PART FIFTH.

THE ART OF FENCING.

CHAPTER I.

THE ART OF FENCING.

Among all physical exercises there is none that gives the body so much strength and skill, as well as certainty, and imparts to all the muscles a more equable movement, and so promotes health, as the art of fencing. It improves the manly form and the expression of the face, and awakens in the young greater energy and caution than they perhaps naturally possess.

Bayonet, spear, and lance do not belong to our domain; we have to do here only with the sword, and indeed only with the rapier (foil).

THRUST FENCING.

To avoid all danger in practice, the real sword is replaced by the foil, the face covered by a wire mask, the hands by well-lined gloves, and the upper body, to which alone all the strokes are directed, protected by a stout jacket, the collar and right side of which are of leather. The foil is a circular or quadrangular rod or blade of pliable, highly tempered steel, thirty-one to thirty-eight inches in length, blunted and covered with leather at the point.

The foil is divided into two parts, *offensive* and *defensive*. The first, measured from the point to the middle, is called the "weak part," and is the offensive part; the second, measured from the middle to the handle, is called the "strong part," and is the defensive part.

The Measure.

When two fencers stand opposite each other ready for conflict, their distance apart is called the *measure*. This is the correct position when the sword-blades cross each other in the midst. The distance is then so great that by a mere extending of the arm, each adversary only touches the breast of the other with the point of his foil, and could only thrust him through by a thrust with the normal sally.

If the rivals stand nearer each other, so that a thrust might take place without the sally, or without any other forward movement, the measure is called *shortened;* and if they stand so far apart that the thrust is possible only by means of an exaggerated sally by a rush or spring, the measure is called *extended.* The fencers stand outside the limits if the distance from each other is greater than that last mentioned.

The breast side of the two fencers is called the *inner;* the back, the *outer*.

If one imagines a middle line of the body from the aggressor and defendant to the feet, and the point here where each touches the ground united to the other by a direct line, this line is the *fencing-line*, and its vertical plane is the normal *fencing-plane*.

Place and Position.

The first movement the beginner has to learn is the fundamental position, known as the *defensive attitude*.

On account of the arm bearing the weapon, this is called the *central* or *primary* position, or more plainly, the *advance*. From this position arise all movements, aggressive and repellent. This attitude consists of two positions : —

First Position.

The pupil takes his place, himself erect with extended knees, the feet at right angles, heel to heel, the right foot, the right side and face turned toward the teacher. The body must be held firm and erect, the arms hanging lightly and easily at the sides, the left hand holding the foil a few inches below the handle. Then he places the right hand across the body, and grasps the handle of the foil as the first movement (see Fig. LXXXI., 1) ; as the second movement, he lifts the foil, holding it with both hands, the hands separating as they rise until the arms extend outward above the head. (Fig. LXXXI., 2, 3.) Here he pauses a little. This is the first defensive position.

Our Physical Gymnastics have taught the pupil to move his arms independently of the body, to expand the chest and throw back the shoulders; a necessity in this position.

Second Position.

To assume the second defensive position, the right arm with the foil falls directly downward until its elbow is raised a little above the waist, the lower arm and the foil standing in an oblique upward direction, so that the point of the foil is on a line with the outward eye of the adversary, or on one between both eyes. The hand meantime lies with the nails upward. In this movement the left arm must pass to the left as far as in Fig. LXXV., so that the

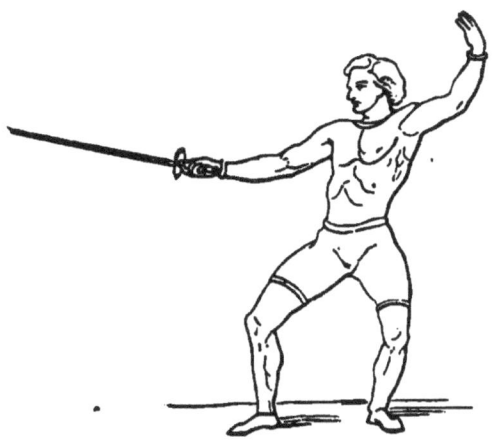

FIG. LXXV.

inner surface of the hand with extended fingers lying close to each other, is turned toward the ear. At the same time, the right foot steps about twenty inches out in the fencing line, and so that the knuckles and knee form a perpendicular line, while the knee of the left leg must extend somewhat beyond the toes of this foot.

In like manner the hip and shoulder lines of the torso, held quite erect and resting upon the left foot, must be exactly within the fencing-plane, and the head be borne erect. The fingers must certainly hold the foil firmly but not convulsively, else weariness may easily ensue, and the finer feeling for action be lost. The index finger, somewhat bent, is placed on one side of the parrying bar, but the thumb is placed on its other side, perpendicularly with the blade, which it still must touch.

These are the two defensive positions which follow in two *tempi*. In this position the fencer receives and gives all thrusts. (Fig. LXXV.)

If, in fencing, there is a sudden transition from right to left, that is, a forward change in defense, one throws quickly the weight of his body upon the foremost foot, turns upon its heel, and brings the hindmost foot and shoulder forward into the fencing-plane, while, at the same moment, he grasps the foil with the left hand, and immediately brings the arm into the right position. If the change of the defense takes place backward, he turns upon the heel of the hindmost foot.

Attitude of the Hand.

The two main attitudes, which the armed hand has to take, are called *primary* (see defensive attitude, Fig. LXXV.) and *secondary*. The first is that already described in the defensive attitude; the latter is the reversed position of the hand, the nails inward, and so secure that the hand at the wrist forms a little angle down-

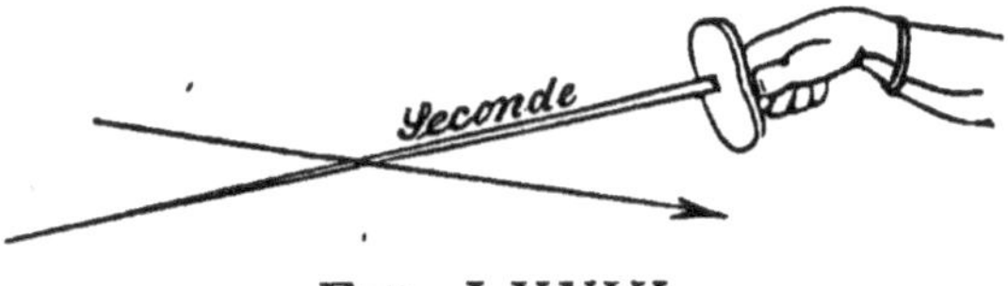

FIG. LXXVI.

ward, the point of the foil being turned downward as much as it is turned upward in the primary position. (Fig. LXXVI.)

Thrusts are always made in these attitudes; for parades there are three other attitudes: (1) The third, in which, as in the second, the nails are turned inward, but the wrist-joint forms no angle downward, but, as in the first, remains with the blade turned outward. (Fig. LXXVII.) (2) The fourth is like the first, only

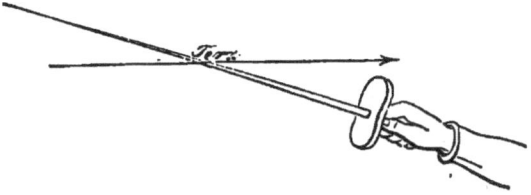

FIG. LXXVII.

the hand-joint forms a slight inner angle. (Fig. LXXVIII.)

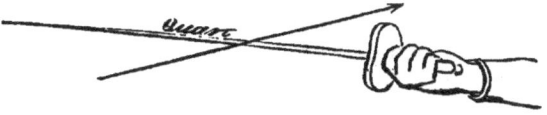

FIG. LXXVIII.

(3) The fifth, like the fourth, with this difference, that the wrist-joint, as in the second, forms a downward angle, and the point of the foil is turned downward. (Fig. LXXIX.)

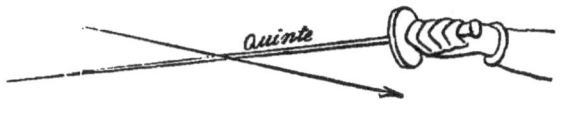

FIG. LXXIX.

As soon as the fencers enter the *measure* opposite each other, they must at once begin the engagement; that is, they must cross blades with edges close but without any mutual pressure, and that upon their inner side.

FENCING MOVEMENTS.

We divide these into foot, arm and weapon movements. (Thrust, parade and feint movements.)

The Foot Movement.

1. The *onset-movement* is a quick raising and a decided setting downward of the foremost foot, several times repeated, while the centre of gravity rests entirely on the firmly placed hindmost foot. Meantime the upper part of the body remains in perfect repose. More belonging to the practice of fencing as a means of attaining a secure defensive position, it also appears in fencing as a means of irritating the adversary; but it must not, as in practice, be a real stamping, but a slight and not too often repeated movement executed only with the toes.

2. The *revolution* takes place with a simultaneous turning of the upper part of the body upon the heel of the hindmost foot, and a swaying of the foremost foot.

3. The *sally* takes place as follows: — The foremost (right) foot takes a rapid step forward, the upper body following unbent while the hindmost (left) foot remains firm but extended in its place. The sally is the most important movement, and very difficult in execution, because a thrust is always connected with it. It is well for pupils to practice it first with the feet, the arms remaining planted in the hips; and to take later the practice for arm-movements, as it will be given in our "Primary Thrust."

The *erect* or *return* movement in the defensive attitude takes place by means of a powerful wrench of the body, a decided drawing back of the foremost and a bending of the hindmost foot, with the upper body erect, following immediately upon a thrust.

In this movement everything depends upon its being performed with *one* stroke, as skill in resuming quickly the defensive attitude enables the fencer to parry in a moment the thrust of his rival, in case his own attack has failed.

4. The step forward and backward (also called the advance), takes place while, without allowing the upper part of the body to lose its defensive attitude, the right foot is shoved forward a hand's breadth, and at the moment when it touches the floor, lets the left foot take its place.

The step backward (also called the retreat) takes place in a reversed way, the rear (left) foot making the first movement toward the rear. The object of these two movements is to gain ground, or to relinquish it without even for a moment losing the defensive attitude. They are also used as *feints* to bring the rival from his place and to deceive him. In practice they are not used often in succession because when a larger ground is covered another step is employed called the *passade*.

5. The *passade* takes place in two *tempi*. At one, the hindmost (left) foot steps a hand's breadth before the foremost (right) foot, while this, turning upon its heel, turns the toes somewhat outward, so that both soles form a right angle. At two, the right foot, remaining exactly in the fencing-line, moves forward a shoulder's breadth, while the left, by a slight turn upon the ball, forms a rectangle at the right, so that the defensive attitude is resumed only a step in front of the original place.

The *passade march* ensues when the *passade* is executed several times in succession. The backward *passade* follows in like manner, only with a reversed movement of the feet.

Facility in all these movements must have been acquired by practice, before passing on to others. The pupil must not become disheartened at their difficulty, for they are the foundation of the art of fencing.

THRUSTS.

Thrusts are primary and secondary ; and these are again divided into backward and forward (or feint thrusts), double and simultaneous. If the one attacked makes a thrust before the aggressor can resume his defensive attitude, it is called an after-thrust. If one of the fencers only outlines a thrust, but makes a real one immediately after, it is called a forward (mock or feint) thrust. Double and simultaneous thrusts are what their name signifies. If one makes a thrust twice in succession without resuming the erect position after the first, it is called a double thrust. Simultaneous thrusts are those when both fencers strike at once.

If the defender, by a mere extending of his arm and weapon, without a sally, lets the hotly advancing assailant rush as it were upon his foil's point, this is called an *arrêt-thrust*.

The thrust will usually delicately graze the rival blade, but there are circumstances when forced thrusts occur in which a hard-onset on the rival blade takes place with a pressure of one's own weapon.

It is customary for rivals to attack in the right side (from within), but there are cases when it is advisable to attack a rival from without (in the left).

Two men standing opposed to each other, must observe at the first glance, that two points of attack stand open to them : namely, the inner space of the sword and the outer, and indeed these only. But in fencing, these are again divided into the points above and below the hand, as well for the outer line as the inner one. This gives four points of onset, or to speak more plainly, four unguarded points upon which the rival can be attacked. To cover these four points, there are four defensive movements, called *parade* movements, of which we shall treat later.

The Primary Thrust.

The primary thrust proceeds immediately from the guard attitude with sally, in the following manner : The right arm, at the moment of the sally, is extended from the height of the shoulder, in a horizontal direction, while the point of the foil is energetically pushed toward the goal. At the same moment when the foremost (the right) foot steps forward and the thrusting movement begins, the left hand falls at the left thigh, still a few inches from it, and the left leg is extended. The foremost (right) side, shoulder, knee and toes, forms a perpendicular line, while the left side, from shoulder to foot, forms a straight, oblique line. (Fig. LXXX.) This thrust is applied to upper as well as inner and outer thrusts.

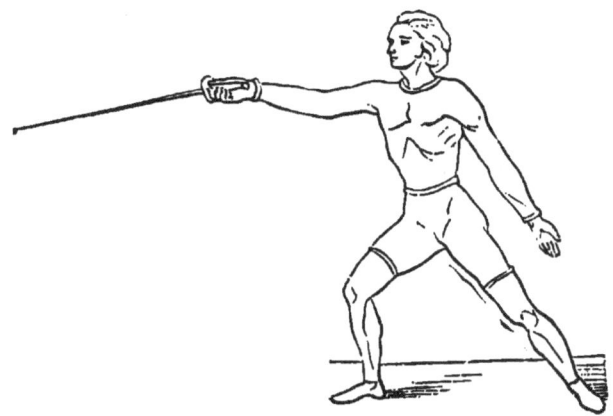

FIG. LXXX.

We have seen in the sally how the erection to the defensive attitude proceeds with the feet and torso; we have to add in relation to the arms: The hindmost (left) arm rises quickly to its required height in the defensive attitude; the foremost (right) is drawn backward quickly, so that the whole body again resumes its defensive attitude.

The pupil will do well to divide, in exercise, the thrust into two *tempi*. At one, extending of the arm; at two, onset. In practice both fall into one *tempo*.

The Secondary Thrust

Consists in extending the arm, a turning of the fist from the primary to the secondary, and sally. This, in practice, again takes place in two *tempi*. This thrust is applied in lower thrusts when the one attacked, holding his fist too high, thereby leaves his lower body unprotected. (See second attitude, Fig. LXXVI.)

The Parades.
Simple Parades.

We have learned, in regard to the thrusts, that there are four unprotected points at which the fencer may be attacked ; to cover these there are four defensive movements called " Parades." As the prime or central attitude deviates from the normal one, above, below, or sideway, the form of the parade will vary ; and the parades are designated as second, third, fourth and fifth. Third and fourth protect against upper, second and fifth against lower, third and second against outward, fourth and fifth against inner thrusts.

The form of the parades depends upon the attitudes of the fist, which we have accurately described. The arm must be extended.

The parades must always be executed firmly and decidedly, but never with a sideward-push of the hostile foil.

Counter-parades.

Every simple parade has its counter-parade. The attitude of the hand is as in the simple parade, only with this difference, that the foil describes a full circle ; that is, at the " counter-fourth " the hand remains in the fourth position, while the weapon, passing down from the inside up to the outside, reaches the place whence it started.

All other counter-parades have the same course ; if we know one we know all.

The feints, in the narrow sense of the word, are only deceptive, specious movements, by which the two-fold contest is carried on ; every fencer seeks to entice his opponent into an uncovered position, prepares, modulates and delivers his thrusts.

The following movements are to be designated and elucidated as feints:
1. The *dégagement* or *dégagé*.
2. The *doublé*.
3. The *coupé*.

1. *The Dégagement.*

In this attack the foil-point of the aggressor sinks under the blade of his rival, and passing close under it, rises on the opposite side; at the same moment his arm is extended and the thrust made. If the thrust is not made, if the foil-point passes at once back the same way to its original position, this is called the *double-dégagé*.

The *dégagement*, simple as well as double, is very often employed, especially in the beginning of fencing, to bother the rival and entice his weapon from the right position.

2. *The Doublé*

Is very simple in its application, but endlessly effective. It differs from the double *dégagé* in this respect: the latter is only a to-and-fro *dégagé*, while the former goes on to complete an entire circle. But this is to be done only when the defendant, after the first *dégagement*, follows in the same direction. If this happens many times, a circling of blades round each other takes place until a thrust follows.

3. *The Coupé.*

Differs from the *dégagé* in this way: The aggressor, instead of thrusting his foil from the inside out under the hostile blade, by bending the fist passes before its point into the *dégagé*.

Compliment of Arms.

It is customary before beginning the sally for the fencers, as well as the seconds, to salute each other. It is done in this way:
After the fencers have taken places opposite each other accord-

ing to the rules laid down, the teacher gives the following commands:—

1. *Present the hand to your adversary!*

While the left hand quietly holds the foil at the side, the fencer with his right, gracefully salutes his rival.

2. *Hand to the sword-handle!*

According to rules for first position (See Fig. LXXXI., 1.)

3. *Draw the weapon over the head!*

As in Fig. LXXXI., 2, 3. The dotted arms over the head.

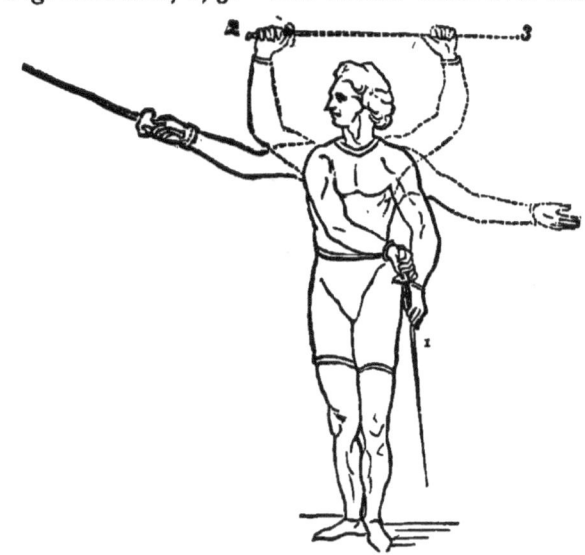

FIG. LXXXI.

4. *Defensive position!*

According to description of second attitude (Fig. LXXV.)

5. *Two appels!*

See Part Fifth, *appel*-step.

6. *Open arms!*

(See Fig. LXXXI. The outstretched, dotted arms.)

7. *Measure, or in line.*

One fencer falls out of line until he almost touches the breast of his rival (See Fig. LXXX.), but with the foil held horizontally. If the rival stands too far away, he steps up to the point ; if he stands too near, he steps, (carefully covering his retreat) backward.

8. *Salute fourth!*

The hand movement of No. 1 will now be made with the foil to the second, toward the outside of the opponent, as in Fig. LXXVIII.

9. *Salute third!*

(See Fig. LXXVII.) To the inner side of the adversary.

10. *Salute both!*

The fencers salute in fourth (Fig. LXXVIII.).

11. *Turn the hand in third!*

The hand is turned from the fourth to the third position. (Fig. LXXVII.)

12. *Ramassement!*

Hands as in Fig. LXXXI., and without pause, drawing the weapon over the head, (Fig. LXXXI, 2, 3.)

13. *Defensive position!* (Fig. LXXV.)

After a longer or shorter salutation the contest begins. These salutes with weapons must be elegantly carried out. The spectator then has the feeling that two really skilful fencers are engaged.

General Advice.

1. Never look at your own foil, but keep a sharp watch over the eye and hand of your antagonist.

2. The foil-point of the aggressor must always be nearer the rival, than the latter's foil-point to him (the aggressor).

3. Attack always at the required distance so that the rival may have no mischance to complain of.

4. Keep always the right line if you would not offer too many exposed points to the rival's sword.

5. After all, the main thing is—cool blood.

PART SIXTH.

MAIN PRINCIPLES OF DRESS.

CHAPTER I.

MAIN PRINCIPLES OF DRESS.

Nature is everywhere harmonious, but the greatest harmony meets us in the human figure. It is, therefore, our task not to distort the form of the human body by dress and adornment, but to allow it to reach its fullest development. Whatever the demands of fashion may be, the finely cultured man or woman may not be absolved from this duty. One will not slavishly follow the mode, but with fine tact take away here, add there, and especially consider what best suits his individuality, and what in color suits his complexion or temperament. To the woman falls a task far more difficult than that of the man; for, while the woman may beautify her appearance, by the cut and arrangement of her dress, by ornaments, ribbons, plumes, and especially by manifold colors, the man of our century is confined to a simple and restricted dress with little choice of color.

Woman's Dress.

We say that the greatest harmony meets us in the human form. Here are symmetry, order, proportion, animated variety, perfect blending of all the parts into one whole. The dress and adornment employed by women can and must have no other purpose than to assist or render more pleasing one or another part of the figure, and they must never detract from the ease of the dress or the entire appearance. Woman should be the emblem of a beautiful simplicity; tasteful, moderate ornament only enhances the charm of this simplicity, while affected, forced, strikingly conspicuous ornament may attract attention, not to loveliness of the form, but to the price and workmanship of the ornaments.

The greatest art in toilet adornment consists in having it in the utmost possible harmony with the person. It would be a great fault, and the lady would miss her aim entirely, if, for instance, a small, charming figure should wear elaborate and carefully arranged ornaments, while they ought to be light and seemingly improvised. On the contrary, a tall, majestic figure may wear to advantage a heavy and elaborate dress. In the toilet self-love and vanity must so far vanish that each one arrives at this conviction: "Nature has made me so and so, and only this suits my face and figure." For the sole office of adornment is to enhance the natural charms, and this may be realized as well through colors as by the form of the clothes, and the ornaments.

A great mistake in women lies in paying entire attention to the adornment of the face and its surroundings, to the neglect of other parts of the body. The face and head certainly form that part upon which the eye of the observer falls first, but the adornment of this part should never destroy the harmony of the whole figure. Above all, the lady must keep before her a decided impression of the whole, with which every single part must harmonize in place and quality. A beautiful face receives the full might of its charm only from beauty of the whole person.

Hence it appears clearly that in dress harmony is far more difficult of attainment than magnificence. The choice of a costume must always be dictated by circumstances. The hostess, by a simple dress, shows that she is ready for our service; costly adornment would not allow us to feel at home in her presence. At the sick bed of a friend, a simple house dress is far more appropriate than an elegant walking costume. In a social gathering more care in dress is required, but a really fine dress is only for festal occasions, such as balls, theatres, concerts, etc. To appear here in ordinary attire would be an open breach of propriety and an insult to the company.

At all religious solemnities, especially at church, the dress must be simple, sober, and modest. We must avoid all that is really adornment, if we would not incur the reproach of decking ourselves in fine array for the house of God. A lady in mourning, whose dress gives evidence of great art and care, will not excite our sympathy. Upon the promenade, as in all circles connected with it, one should appear in a costume which holds a medium between a house dress and a grand toilet,—which, while it displays care and some degree of ornament, is removed from all stiffness and constraint.

Various ages and conditions require varied dress. The young girl, who has just become a bride, must modify somewhat the dress that so charmingly became her as a young maiden, if she would impress us as an amiable wife. Her dress must still show a desire to give her beauty its full value, but never to attract attention. With increasing years, colors and forms should become more quiet. No sight is more ridiculous than that of an elderly lady seeking to represent youth in dress and demeanor. Every period of life has its various appropriate and charming forms and colors, and the woman's task is to select the most fitting, and to confess to herself that it is time to choose them. If a beautiful woman neglects this, she will never attain the end she desires.

All peoples and all eras have given great care to the adornment of the head; this has been especially the case with women, who in this way have great transformations at command. But a lady must not allow herself to be so carried away by a fashion, as to adopt it merely because it is the fashion without considering whether or not it harmonizes with her face. The main thing in the woman's head-gear is to harmonize the reigning mode with the natural form of the face.

The long face demands smooth hair over the forehead, falling on both sides in thick curls; but the round face requires the hair worn high above the forehead, in some becoming form, the ears being left wholly uncovered. A short, broad face gains by having the hair still more drawn back, and also by having it waved, as both modes make the face appear less short and broad. It is also advisable to wear the hair drawn back from the forehead when it grows too low down, and gives the forehead a narrow appearance. A long face appears still longer and more plain if the hair is drawn back or piled up over the forehead ; a broad face, on the contrary, only wins by this mode. Attention to other people's ways of arranging the hair, unprejudiced observation and analysis of each part of this adornment, and then a critical survey of her own before the mirror,—this is the practical school in which the cultured and tasteful lady may make speedy and visible progress in the art of a fine toilet. If, through repeated effort, she has found an arrangement of the hair suited to her face, she may prize it as a real means of enhancing her beauty, and she will not merely for fashion's sake hasten to exchange it for another, perhaps less becoming mode. The mode, which really enhances her beauty of face and figure, she should regard as her own mode, and, holding fast to it, never change it save in trifles.

An indispensable condition of the head-dress is airiness and movement, with an avoidance of all pretension. Ribbons and veils must be light and fluttering. If a lady chooses plumes for the adornment of her head, they must never be stiff, but float lightly and gracefully. One avoids placing ribbons and jewels or metals and feathers together, as also adding long feathers to veils. If ornamental pins and combs for the hair are not to be regarded as tawdry finery, they must be always real, or concealed by ribbons, veil or curls. Bright colors should be removed from the face by a proper arrangement of the hair, or they will detract from its beauty. As for the form of the lady's hat, there is no doubt that the round, graceful form, which displays the whole outline of the head, is preferable to the exaggerated, puffed-up form.

Men's Dress.

Although the fashion of our century does not allow a man the variety in dress and its adornment which is permitted to women, he must be none the less careful in the choice of materials, colors and forms. Clumsy boots or shoes, or a coarse, ill-formed hat spoils the finest toilet. Let the form of the hat be elegant, and always suited to the face. A low hat better suits long, thin faces, than a high one; small faces are also seen at a disadvantage under high or broad-brimmed hats. Almost any form is suited to full faces, but the high hat more so than the low one. The hat must not sit near the eye-brows; still less far from them. The latter may all too easily become ridiculous. Caps are allowed only in the house or on journeys, and do not belong to men's toilet.

In dressing the neck it must be taken into account whether the neck is long, short, thick or thin. In the first case, it must be dressed higher, in the second, lower, in the third, thinner, in the last, thicker.

We have said that men must pay due regard to material, form and color, which, taken as a whole, must be suited to individuality, age and condition. For the man of culture, the use in view decides — show and ornament being entirely subordinate. All over-dressing is especially to be avoided. A costly but not too showy breast-pin, two genuine rings at most, are his ornaments. Fine, white linen is, above all, a sign of good taste and cleanliness.

The form of the dress-coat always follows the reigning mode, and can deviate from it only in trifling respects. The color of the coat is always black on festal occasions; for walking or for morning visits, etc., it may be brown or blue. Nearly all colors may be chosen for the coat. Whether a white or black vest shall be worn with a black dress-coat, depends upon the ruling mode. The pantaloons are subject to the constant changes of fashion; not too wide or too narrow is the best rule here. In regard to this article of dress it may be observed that if colored it should always be lighter than the coat.

The gloves must be of fine leather and sit well; white for festal occasions, light brown, yellowish, or ash gray for every-day wear. As in the pantaloons, one has to consider here that the gloves must be lighter than the coat. Ash-gray and fawn-color are well suited to every dark colored coat; black or dark gloves must never be worn with a light costume. One wears glasses only when he really needs them. The frames should be of gold or silver. The man of culture will only carry the glasses to the eyes when really necessary; a continual adjusting of them to the eyes is silly. Watch chains should always be genuine; if such an one cannot be had, one wears his watch suspended from a simple black ribbon.

In the choice of colors the man should pay careful regard to his face, hair and figure. Black, brown, dark blue and steel-green suit every face; light blue, light gray, fawn-color, and similar hues, are becoming only to fresh, animated faces, and brown hair.

All we have said refers just as much to the dress of the actor as to that of the private man. Still some remarks must be added for the benefit of the former.

If cleanliness, neatness and good form in dress are especial obligations of the cultured man, the actor is doubly bound by these obligations; not because thousands of eyes rest upon him, but because he is to serve as a pattern, because the stage should be the school of culture and fine manners, and an offence against them here deserves to be far more strictly punished. Above all, the actor must avoid appearing upon the stage in the dress in which the public is wont to see him on the street. It makes an unpleasant impression when we think of a Mr. So-and-So, and he appears to us in the person of the actor So-and-So. Even if the audience are not so deceived as to be unaware that the actor Mr. X. plays this or that rôle, they must, under no condition, be reminded of it by the street dress of the actor. But here it is by no means said that the actor is to wear no part of his street costume upon the stage; he is only reminded that he must not appear in his entire street dress, which in itself forms a decided whole, before the eyes of the public, which would then see another character than that of the actor.

In regard to dress that is not modern, and that in stage language is designated by the word "costume," it conforms strictly to the time in which the persons represented lived ; and if we understand how to represent the historical costume correctly, we might still warn against a too strict truth to history ; that is, we would advise the player to adopt the historical costume only so far as decorum, custom and the law of beauty allow.

Ladies will do well to consult their associates over the choice of colors, so that not two or three persons may appear in the same colors, if it is not especially necessary. It is also to be observed that in characters whose main trait is ease, new costumes, which are always stiff, are not to be chosen; neither in characters which portray old age, niggardliness, avarice, etc.

Combination of Colors.

In conclusion we will make some remarks upon colors and their combinations.

Colors are usually divided into primary or purely fundamental colors — yellow, red and blue ; into secondary, which are formed by two primary colors,— orange from yellow and red, green from yellow and blue, purple from red and blue ; and finally tertiary colors, of which there also three, and which always result from the combination of two secondary colors, in which one color rules: — citron-yellow from green and orange ; reddish brown from orange and purple ; and, finally, olive-green from a mixture of purple and green. Besides, we have half-neutral tints : brown, maroon (like the color of the Italian chestnut), and gray ; last of all the neutral tints, white and black.

The fewer colors in one and the same toilet, the more tasteful it is. White and black are always the best and noblest hues for dress, singly as well as in their combinations.

For pale faces, yellow, light blue and pale blue, violet and light gray are to be avoided ; and a brownish, sallow complexion in either sex always appears to disadvantage in white, yellow, light gray, and especially pale, light colors.

Here becoming dark colors must be chosen. Black, dark or steel-green, dark blue, crimson, dark gray and brown, must here in the toilet be blended with white. These colors are becoming to almost every face, but in florid complexions, crimson, bright red and reddish brown are to be avoided. On the contrary, light gray, fawn-color, and even light green, like very light-colored dresses, for the most part are well suited to lively, fresh and brunette faces. For brunette ladies, yellow and red are becoming in hatbands as well as in clothing. Blondes, on the contrary, should avoid all yellow shades, and turn to delicate green, rose and lilac, which colors are in turn less becoming to brunette faces.

Black, white, sky-blue, rose-red, and straw are the noblest colors. Then come those most intimately related to them. The contrasting colors are : green and pink, silver and yellow, black and brown, violet and yellow, blue and orange, rose and light green. The harmonizing colors are : black and pale yellow; sky-blue to white and pale yellow; blue to white; pale blue and pale rose-red; black to white; to scarlet and lilac only white, silver and pale straw; to dark brown, white and straw; crimson and blue; sea-green and yellow ; red and gold ; black and gold ; also black, red and gold ; gold and silver ; silver and blue ; red, brown and lilac ; yellow and lilac ; yellow, brown, black and red ; green and red ; brown, yellow, red, blue and broken gray and black tones ; yellow and black ; white and yellow ; yellow, white and gray ; red and black ; red and yellow ; lilac, blue and red ; white and green ; white and rose ; white and yellow ; in short, white with all colors.

Blondes should choose delicate colors and those blending in combination ; brunettes, on the contrary, contrasting and independent colors, such as bright red and brown, bright yellow and violet, flame-color and black. White stuffs, such as linens, laces and silks, should never affect bluish, but rather yellowish tints, if they are to harmonize with the color of the flesh. If the complexion has greenish or grayish tints, dark green or dark gray may be worn, but here black is preferable.

The brightest colors should, so far as possible, always be next to the head and face ; loud and contrasting ones should be divided and not brought into too great masses. Hence it follows that they are not to be used for the main color of the dress, but only for its decoration. All dark colors' should, if practicable, be arranged below and light ones uppermost. Shoes of very light color should never be worn with dark or black dresses ; red, pink or yellow ones should not be chosen ; but light colored shoes are suited to light toilets.

A toilet of entire white, with even ribbons and ornaments corresponding, is uncommonly delicate, betrays a fine, noble taste, and is suited to august occasions. For joyous festivals, a garniture of rose, sky-blue, pale green, or delicate leaves and flowers, is an agreeable innovation. For elderly persons, black is incontestably not only the most suitable, but also the most dressy ; next to this are fine browns, blue or gray, as best suits the complexion. Colors destined for evening toilets should be chosen by artificial light.

PART SEVENTH.

Application of the Rules Given in this Book to Common Life, the Salon and the Stage.

CHAPTER I.

APPLICATION OF THE RULES GIVEN IN THIS BOOK TO COMMON LIFE, THE SALON AND THE STAGE.

As we have hitherto given only fundamental rules, and in them have regarded people only from the stand-point of æsthetic gymnastics, so shall we now, in the application of the rules laid down, fix only main principles, as we allow man to pass before us in his social relations.

What is Decorum?

One who has thus far studied our book carefully, can be in no doubt as to the answer to this question. But the dramatic artist must be interested in having this word *decorum* somewhat further elucidated. And who in this matter can be considered better authority than our old master, Iffland? We therefore let him speak for himself:

" By the term *decorum* many actors think of nothing but especially distinguished manners. They think to attain them by a lofty carriage of the head, by a measured gait, by a vacant stare which sees and recognizes nothing. They, therefore, choose the most high-stepping, magnificent figure that occurs to them as the ideal of fine manners. They should rather say to themselves —good manners are that deportment which the person to be represented would naturally assume in the given situation.

" The deportment of the prince, of the minister, the general, the rich man, the father, if each is a man of culture, must, in the main, be more or less the same. In some cases, professional habits and costume may change the outward appearance. Temperament, character, and passion must also necessarily produce differences in deportment. The ordinary dancing-master cannot give this instruction. The genius, the peculiarities of the actor must be his inspiration.

"Those who have not received early instruction in fine manners, and must rely wholly upon later instruction, will at least seek to grasp fundamental rules, and try to adapt themselves fully to the requirements of good breeding. This is possible, when the feeling for beautiful forms is especially decided.

"To acquire manifold ideas on this subject, it is excellent to see distinguished men at moments when they are conspicuously before the world, or may be supposed to be in peculiar states of mind. Even if they do not possess the gift of outward representation, still, at such moments, their manners are controlled by the predominant idea, and from the way in which they pass through the ceremonial, one learns to perform decidedly what is necessary.

"It is not in the power of every one to acquire fine manners. It is given to but few. It is, however, granted to many to attain a good deportment. Yet no one can excuse himself if a decent one be wanting.

"This can be attained by ordinary attention. Nothing more retards its attainment than those negligences one allows one's self in every day life, and especially at home. The actor should at all times demean himself as if opposite the *parterre*."

Politeness and Modesty.

"Be polite to every one, whether he stands above or below you," is a common maxim which must be made the main principle of every person who pretends to culture. By politeness we do not understand cringing to others. Let each one ask himself in all cases (if in doubt over the degree of politeness), how he would wish others to meet him, and the doubt will at once vanish. If politeness does not spring from the deepest depths of one's nature, it has the contrary effect, for nothing is more repulsive than politeness that arises from cool and deliberate calculation. It is impossible to give exact, exhaustive rules; he who has a sincere desire to be polite will always find rules; but general hints may certainly be given.

The polite man will regard each individuality from its own standpoint, and give it its full value as such; he will take it as it is, and not as it should be. He will not seek forcibly to impress his own ideas upon others; he will represent them merely as his own, and not as general and irrefutable. If he is not questioned, he is silent; if he is questioned, he gives his opinion plainly, but in the most inoffensive way. This manner is far more effective than the domineering one, and not in the least derogatory to politeness.

It is impolite to interrupt one when speaking, without urgent reasons, or to remark that his recitals do not wholly agree with facts. If the departure is slight, one is entirely silent; if it is so marked that harm might ensue, one begs pardon, and remarks that the narrator may not have been quite correctly informed, and correct the error in such a manner as not to wound. In like manner, if the honor and reputation of a person not present are attacked, politeness never decrees silence, but to a manly defense of the one unjustly assailed.

The polite man never omits the required greeting; he does not wait anxiously for the first greeting from him he meets; if not directly anticipating him he at least approaches half way, and never omits the salutation, or to recognize it, even if it comes from the lowest. It is impolite not to give the best possible information in reply to a question; if want of time or knowledge of the matter do not allow an exact answer, an excuse must follow, but never must bad humor or ill-will be evident in the reply. Any one may be betrayed into a breach of politeness; but it would be in the highest degree impolite not to offer an immediate apology.

Many people gauge their own politeness by that of others; this is entirely false. Our politeness should not be decided by outside things; it must come from within, and we should not permit ourselves to be less polite because another is impolite. It is unworthy of any one to repress his inward convictions out of politeness, merely for the sake of flattering another. It is impolite to allow any one to remark that he is not intellectually our equal. If one is at the same time pretentious and ignorant, long conversation with him is to be avoided in society; by a display of intellectual superiority, one usually more offends the host and the company than the person himself whom he would humiliate.

To make a timid, bashful man ridiculous in society by perpetrating witticisms at his expense, is not only impolite—it is execrable. Such conduct has often had a decided effect for life upon the unfortunate individual, by depriving him of every remnant of self-confidence.

Modesty must be united with politeness. The modest man should be well conscious of his worth, but not to make a display of it, still less to look down upon less favored persons.

A really able but forward man lowers the measure of his ability, while the modest man heightens it. Modesty, like politeness, must proceed from the heart; if it is only assumed and outward, it may easily make the contrary impression of arrogance upon those around us. In like manner we must warn against too great modesty when it goes so far as to wholly forget one's own interests, even to neglect them, from too high a sense of honor or the wish to serve others.

So much of modesty and of politeness in general,—that dictated by the heart (for in our book we have nothing to do with the politeness of the diplomatist). Special things will be learned under single headings in the course of this part.

Behavior Upon the Street and Public Places in the Open Air.

The man of culture does not meditate upon the street; he does not walk dreamily forward with hands crossed over his back, eyes cast upon the ground; he does not pause from time to time; he goes on his way, not arrogantly, but with firm step, his glance straight forward, yet so that he can see what happens in front of him and at his side. If he meets a person of his own rank, he salutes, turning half aside; if he meets a lady, he steps aside far enough to permit her to pass freely; if the path is narrow, he pauses, and lets the lady go past him; in bad weather, he always steps aside and gives the lady the better path. Salutation upon the street takes place by removing the hat at least three steps in front of the person to be saluted, and ends three steps behind him. (How we have learned under "Salutation.") The removal of the hat will begin earlier or later, according to the rank of the person greeted. A premature removal of the hat is no sign of great respect; on the contrary, it is ridiculous.

The manner of pausing before every acquaintance, and without any special reason, engaging him in conversation, is not that of the cultivated man. In most cases one salutes in passing, but if he meets a prince, he steps aside, pauses, and remains standing with uncovered head until he is past. If in walking one chances to glance upward and observes a person at a window, he bows; but to glance persistently right and left into open windows, and seize every possible opportunity of bowing, does not belong to fine tone.

If a group stand conversing upon the street, every one of this group turns fully to the side whence the greeting comes; if this does not happen, if one stands quietly in his place, and bows as it were over the shoulder, he commits a breach of good manners. If one passes through a dividing and larger group, and must bow on both sides, until past, he carries his hat at the side of the thigh.

There are people who lay great stress upon being greeted (recognized), for this reason none should neglect it. Just as little should one omit to have the same degree of respect in the greeting returned as in that given. It evidences little culture to return a polite greeting indifferently or coldly.

If we accompany any one who salutes a stranger to us, politeness demands that we bow also, and in like manner that we return the bow if our companion is greeted. But if our companion is a person of higher rank than we ourself, we do not return the bow which is for him alone.

Ladies must pay great attention to their street deportment. What in men may pass for ill-breeding or lack of culture, may easily assume a worse character in women. Hence they should avoid all unnecessary gazing around, when passing along the street; still, anxiety must not cause a lady to neglect to return the greetings she receives with a polite bow. (See Reverence in Walking). The lady never bows first,* but if she receives a bow, she must in all cases return it. Most mothers believe they have educated their daughters remarkably well, if they pass with short, tripping steps over the street, glancing neither right nor left so as not to be obliged to return salutations too often, which would be improper. Into what an error are they betrayed! The woman, conscious of her worth, conscious that she serves as a pattern of morals, may walk on freely and unaffectedly, not allowing the least anxiety or embarrassment to be remarked in her glance or bearing. Thus only she avoids that which through an anxious manner she had thought to shun.

Deportment Toward Ladies.

Let one adopt what we have said in regard to Politeness and Modesty, and he will have the rule for his deportment toward ladies. We will add a few things.

As politeness must be dictated by the heart, so must the deportment toward ladies be devoid of everything superficial or forced; a clever woman distinguishes very sharply between flattery and truth. We never rise in the respect of women by a pretense of kindly service. A worthy complaisance is the required condition.

---

* In America, the lady always bows first. She thereby gives the gentleman permission to bow to her.

Always, and in all situations, ladies are given the preference; but in mounting a stair-case, propriety demands that the gentleman precede the lady, and upon reaching the top wait at one side the stairs, until the lady is also at the top, and then take his place at her side or behind her.

The man of culture and tact never, in presence of a lady, leads the conversation to pure science, politics or religion, or to any domain where the lady may not safely follow. If the lady herself begins such a conversation, he proceeds with great circumspection, continuing only so long as it is the lady's pleasure to follow, which, with due attention, he remarks at once. A man in ladies' society must be very careful about remarks upon beauty, ugliness or age; nowhere can he give greater offense than here. If a man has cause and occasion to pay one lady marked respect in the presence of others, this must not be carried so far as to outrage common respect toward the others. A woman seldom forgives this, and the one thus distinguished may easily be thrown into embarrassment. In the society of ladies the man never belongs especially to one individual, but to the whole. If he will not, or thinks he cannot observe this rule, he had better remain away from society.

A merry humor is always welcome in the society of ladies, but this must never pass permitted limits, neither must the tone of the conversation be too loud or too familiar. If a lady seats herself on a sofa, and invites a gentleman to be seated, but does not make an unmistakable motion for him to take a place on the sofa, he draws a chair near it, and seats himself upon that.

Deportment in Large Companies.

When the gentleman enters the hall, he goes immediately to the lady of the house, pays her his first compliments, the master of the house his second, and then to the others present. Politeness demands that among the latter, persons of rank be saluted first. It scarce need be hinted that these greetings must be short, no especial pause being made at either, least of all before the host and hostess. If the lady of the house is not in the first room, the person entering, passes, with a slight bow to those present, into the next room, seeking her, to salute her; then only does he mingle with the company.

The guest must notice carefully whether upon his entrance the lady or the master of the house is in conversation with other guests; in this case, he waits a favorable opportunity before approaching, so as not to interrupt the conversation.

If, for the guest, the society is made up of many strange elements, he must gradually be introduced to one and another, by an acquaintance. One acquaintance leads to another, and thus initiation takes place. Regarding the principle that in society every single person belongs to the whole, one will avoid all marked isolation, whether from individuals or from the many. Single, greater or smaller groups must needs form, but they should not be of long duration; they should soon dissolve and the individual members again blend with others.

If, in a company, recitations or performances are given by professional artists, the laity will do well not to undertake them; but if on the contrary, everyone does his best, no one who has the capability of entertaining the company in any way, may excuse himself.

We would here especially warn against one very frequent and obtrusive piece of ill-breeding; this is the want of attention when one or another person performs something. Conversation between individuals should cease at once, and if one finds no pleasure in the performance, he must never let his dissatisfaction be visible in any way. Unhappily, we find this breach of good manners in the most refined circles. How constantly we see two or more persons during the performance of a piece on the piano, engaged in animated conversation, thus gaining more or less the ill-will of the company, and especially that of the performer! All at once as soon as the music ceases, we see and hear them applauding with all their might, and far more lavishly than the most attentive listeners! One can regard such people only with aversion. They show that they are present only for their own sake and not for that of the company.

In introductions it is to be strictly observed that the lower is to be introduced to the higher, the younger to the older, the gentleman to the lady; hence the name and station of the former is always first to be mentioned, and then the name of the one to whom he is introduced. In the case of persons of distinguished rank who are supposed to be generally known, only the name and station of the one introduced, is mentioned.

If one takes a glass, a cup, or any vessel that has contained refreshments from the hand of a lady, he does not set it down in the first place that offers, in which case it may easily be broken; he motions to a servant, and gives it to him. In case no servant is near at the moment, he holds the object in hand until a servant arrives.

If one is engaged in conversation, and a new comer appears, he does not break off the conversation. In a few brief words, he explains its import to the newcomer, and goes on. Secrets which the one just entering may not hear, do not belong to society.

If one seats himself beside one or more persons, immediately before setting down he makes a slight bow to one or all.

Deportment at a Ball.

Deportment at a ball does not differ from deportment in a large company, or from that toward ladies in general. There are still some details to be observed, which we will designate in a few words :—

1. Two successive dances are never danced with one lady.
2. Too frequent dancing with one lady is to be avoided.
3. Politeness demands that we do not always dance only with the ladies who please us, but with those who are less pleasing to us.
4. If a gentleman would invite a lady to dance, he does not gaze around the hall in such a way as to attract attention;

he does not pass by various ladies with a half-air of wishing to engage them; but, from the place where he stands, he singles out his partner, and approaches her with decided steps. One to two steps (according to space) before the lady, the bow is made, and the address follows. In withdrawing from a lady, who is already engaged, he takes a step backward, and withdraws with a bow. It is very impolite if, in this case, he without delay, engages the lady sitting next, which is as much as to say: "Because I cannot have this one, I take you." No greater offense toward a lady is possible. It is better to go back to one's place, and single out another lady, approaching her as the first. It also shows little culture when the gentleman with whom the lady declines to dance, gives evidence of wounded feelings; if the lady is engaged, he has no reason; if she refuses to dance with him for other reasons, the lady fond of dancing has already punished herself, since she must remain sitting at least during this dance, for no lady of culture, after she has given a gentleman a refusal of one dance, will grant this dance to another.

If there is no other reason than that the lady is engaged, politeness demands that in refusing, she begs the hand of the gentleman for the next or for a future dance. If the lady is ready for the dance, she rises immediately upon receiving the invitation; at the same time, the gentleman with one step passes to her left side, and receives in his right hand the finger-tips of the lady's left hand, and with lifted arm steps with her to the place where the dance is to begin. It is impolite to take the lady by the arm as soon as the engagement takes place; it implies a familiarity which must never be displayed at a ball, unless it is a family ball. If the dancing pair have to begin the dance at the very place where the engagement is made, the gentleman after he receives the lady's hand, assumes the proper position and begins.

5. During the dance one avoids every too near approach,

every placing the chin upon the lady or gentleman's shoulder, (a sin against decorum unhappily of frequent occurrence in our day, but especially to be condemned), and pursues the dance in the most well-bred manner, to its close. As soon as the dance is ended, the gentleman leads the lady, in the same way as before beginning it, to her place. Two or three steps before reaching the place, the lady turns to her partner, a slight bow from both takes place, which the lady, now loosing her hand, follows with a full reverence, while the gentleman makes the "reverence at departure."

6. It is especially ill-bred during the ball (except at table,) to draw off the glove, and immediately before or even during the engaging, draw it on again. The man of fine feeling takes two pairs of gloves with him to every ball, and changes as soon as is necessary ; to offer the lady one's hand with a soiled glove on it is indelicate in the highest degree.

7. To come to a ball promised beforehand for all the dances, places the lady in no agreeable position in regard to the gentlemen ; it is well enough to be engaged for two or at the most three dances in advance, but it is not well for a lady to be forced to refuse every gentleman who comes to engage her. Aside from the consideration that it cannot be pleasant for them, it may easily give such a lady the reproach of prudery.

8. At a ball every pair has the same rights ; one should not therefore press into the foreground.

9. In round dances a too rapid movement out of the row of dancers, and dancing in front of it, is ill-bred.

10. The main rule for the cultured man, is to follow implicitly the arrangements of the director of the ball.

11. A dancer has to observe the greatest caution if, during a brief pause, he would say a few words to his lady. If he broaches a grave topic, he bores ; if he speaks superficially, he gives the impression of an effeminate man. He, therefore, well considers with whom he dances, and what he can possibly say.

All we have thus far said in regard to the ball, refers certainly to the first, most refined circles; and it is evident that modifications enter according to the sphere in which the ball takes place; but the man of culture makes no distinction; he remains equally himself everywhere. A man will never incur the reproach of too great refinement, but more often quite the contrary.

Deportment at Table.

In going to the table, the lady of the house and the highest guest take precedence; and when these are seated the others (ladies first) sit down, making a slight bow to the left and right.

Each guest, without further delay, will take the designated place. One takes care not to let it be remarked that he would prefer another place; it is an insult to the hostess and the person near whom he is seated. If one has to choose his own place, he waits modestly until the older and higher in rank are seated.

If the dishes are not handed by a servant, but pass from the lady of the house, a guest always hands the viands to the one next him. It is impolite to break the succession in order to do honor to any single person, by passing the dish to the other side of the table, and then taking it back. On the other hand, it is not only proper, but politeness demands that the dish be held for the lady, until she has helped herself.

If all the dishes have not been passed around, and some still remain upon the table, one does not begin to eat, until the lady or gentleman of the house, or the most distinguished guest, has begun.

Although the rules for sitting have been exactly given in "Æsthetic Gymnastics," a few more words are required here in regard to sitting at table. Here, certainly, the position of the feet is not so strictly subject to rule; but they should never be so stretched out as to annoy one's neighbor opposite. In like manner, it is not allowable to protrude the elbows; they should be so sharply drawn in, that placing them upon the table would be an impossibility.

Meat is to be severed from the bone by knife and fork ; to gnaw at the bone is in the highest degree unmannerly. Bones, as well as those parts of fruit which are not eatable (stones, etc.), belong to the edge of the plate, but the knife and fork upon the knife-rest at its side. After eating soup, the spoon remains in the plate. If the knives are not changed, one cleanses his own with a bit of bread, which, in any event, he lets lie upon his plate.

One does not let the stones of fruit fall from his mouth upon the plate, for in this case there is danger of their springing upon the table-cloth or upon his neighbor's plate ; but one carries his spoon or fork to the lips, places the stone upon it and then carries it to the edge of the plate.

Tarts and cakes are never taken with the fingers, but with a knife ; but comfits (dry ones) are taken with two fingers (the thumb and index finger), and preserved fruits with the spoon.

If one has to pour out wine or water, he does so at the right with the left, and at the left with the right hand.

If at table, one has to reach any sort of thing (spoon, knife fork, glass, bread, etc.) to the lady near him, he never does this with the bare hand, but upon a plate.

A gentleman's first duty certainly is attention to the lady he takes to the table ; but this should never be directed so exclusively to her that he vouchsafes no word to the lady on his left. The man of culture will engage alternately both ladies in conversation.

In eating soup, when the plate begins to be empty, one takes especial care not to strike the spoon audibly against it.

It is very impolite, in helping one's self from a dish, to hold it critically in the hand, and perhaps lay down a piece already touched by the fork, doubtful which to take. If one helps the lady next to him, he should always take the best for her.

One eats meat by cutting off each mouthful separately ; to cut the whole into bits beforehand is exceedingly ill-bred.

One guards against laying knife or fork from the dish which is being carried around upon his own plate ; and one never takes anything from the dish with his own fork ; but in case a fork is lacking, he asks for one from the servant.

One does not cut the roll of bread ; he breaks it.

If a dish is brought on with which one is not acquainted, and which he has never tasted, if he cannot trust his gift for observation and see at a glance how the others do, he lets it pass by him, rather than make himself ridiculous by eating it in the wrong way.

One should be sparing of toasts. The first belongs to the master of the house, while welcoming the company. The highest of the guests returns thanks, by proposing a toast to the master and mistress of the house. If one does not possess the gift of ready speech (which is no demerit), he should not press himself urgently into a reply to a toast, as this may lay him open to ridicule.

The person of highest rank in the company always gives the signal for rising from the table ; often it is the host or hostess. It is in the highest degree ill-mannered to rise before the signal is given.

In rising one makes a slight bow to right and left, and, as in coming to the table, offers his arm to his lady, and conducts her back to the dancing-hall or into another room.

Deportment at the Theatre or Concert.

At the theatre, as in the concert-room, the same rules for deportment are observed as in good society. We have, therefore, only a few remarks to add to what has already been said.

It is especially impolite and contrary to all decorum and culture, to rise too early at the close of a performance, or to begin to prepare for departure by a putting on of wraps, shawls or hats (with ladies). In this way the close of the piece is ruined for the rest of the audience as well as for the performers.

The Visit of Ceremony.

Many reasons give occasion for this visit. Among them are: The rendering of thanks, the conveying of some sort of tidings, congratulations to superiors, requests for promotion, presentation to those dwelling in a house to which one has himself just removed, etc.

If we would enter a room in which we are a stranger, we knock lightly but decidedly on the outside door, and wait for "come in!" If this does not follow, we knock a second time; if no response then comes, we do not enter; we withdraw unless a servant is near from whom we may receive information.

If a servant is at hand, we allow ourselves to be announced; the servant opens the door; and, after we have left in the ante-room, all such objects as cloak, overcoat, cane, umbrella, etc., we enter hat in hand, wearing gloves, which on such occasions we never lay aside, unless the master or mistress of the house request a longer stay, in which case the gloves are removed. Ladies (if the visit is not to a high personage) do not lay aside their hats and cloaks.

If a servant does not open the door, we open it ourself, according to the rules given. (See "Opening of a Door.")

If we enter an empty room in which we are to await the person visited, we remain quietly standing. To go around the room, peering at pictures and furniture, leaning against the latter, opening and gazing into the books lying upon the table, as if testing things, is the height of ill-breeding. The one awaited appears, we approach within a few steps of him, with a bow, then wait to act as he does. If he remains standing, we do the same; if he has a chair set for us, or points to a chair and takes a seat himself, we also take a chair, according to the prescribed rules, seat ourself with a slight bow, and in a few words, make known our errand.

When the visit is over, we take leave in the prescribed way. (See "Opening of the Door upon Leaving.") If we have set the chair ourself, we return it to its former place. (See "Setting Back a Chair.")

If several persons are already in the room with the one to whom the visit is paid, all rise when the master and mistress do so, and remain standing before their chairs until invited to sit down again. If the one to whom the visit is paid is absent, the visitor gives his card to the servant with a corner turned down; if there are several persons to visit, a card must be left for each, with this distinction, that the ladies only leave cards for the ladies of the house, but the gentlemen for both the ladies and gentlemen.

Audience with Princes.

The one entering steps, with hat in his right hand, after the door has opened to him, two or three steps, according to space, into the chamber or hall, and immediately upon the fourth step pays his compliments, naturally, in the most dignified and reverential way. After drawing himself erect, he pauses, his glance fixed upon the prince in deferential expectation. If the prince motions to him to step nearer, he passes to a respectful distance (three steps), makes a second bow, and pauses in silence. One never speaks until the prince requests it. Then he tells his errand briefly and clearly.

When the prince gives a signal that the audience is ended, the visitor makes the Reverence at Departure, goes sideward-backward toward the door, his glance turned to the prince. When he reaches the door, he makes a second bow, and leaves the hall.

During the interview his glance is fixed steadily, but without presumption, upon the prince.

If the prince enters the room when the one who has begged the audience is already there, the latter, as soon as the former enters, makes the first bow, and waits until the prince beckons him to approach or himself approaches. If the prince steps nearer, the visitor makes the second bow on the spot.

If some one enters a hall, in which the prince and princess, as well as the court-circle are present, the first bow is to the prince, the second to the princess.

In coming, as in going, no notice is taken of the others present. In going, the first bow is to the prince, the second to the princess, but at the door only one bow is made.

If the prince approaches some one in the hall and wishes to speak with him, the latter makes a bow at once. The same when the prince leaves him.

It is of service to the dramatic delineator to know that those around the prince, never bow when he is saluted, excepting when a person of higher rank than they themselves enters ; then they bow without waiting for his salutation.

CONCLUSION.

The Manner of Studying this Book without a Teacher.

If the pupil has a teacher, he will prescribe rules ; if the pupil wishes to instruct himself there are only two methods in which this may be done.

The first is : To execute all the movements of Physical and Æsthetic Gymnastics before a large mirror, and in the following way : one does not take position while gazing into the mirror ; he takes it in accordance with his own idea, retains it for a time, and then gazes into the mirror to see if it is right.

The second method we propose to the pupil is far better. Every one has a congenial friend who wishes in some sort to share in this study. With this friend, he begins in the following way : The friend takes the book in hand, seats himself opposite the one who is practising, and while the latter goes through with the prescribed movements, the former observes and criticises what he sees. Then both exchange parts : the critic becomes the pupil and vice versa.

This is the best manner of reaching the desired goal in a short time and in the most direct way.

ERRATA.

The reader will please note the following misprints which have escaped correction. A slight use of the pen or knife will, in most cases, rectify the errors without much defacement of the page :

Page 13, last line, for imperfect word read *clavicle*.

Page 32, first line, for the present sentence read : *From the forward inclination of the head we pass to the left side, to the back, to the right side and again to the forward movement, repeating the whole exercise in reversed order, the upper part of the body*, etc.

Page 44, 9th line, for " LXVII " read *LXVI*.

Page 61, 19th line, for " finger " read *fingers*.

Page 62, 8th line, for " LXVII " read *LXV*.

Page 66, 18th line, for " LXVIII, *a* " read *LXVII, a*.

Page 67, 6th line, for " LXVIII, *a* " read *LXVII, a*.

Page 68, 10th line, for " LXVIII, *a, a* " read *LXVII, a, a*.

Page 83, 8th line, for " LXXVIII " read *LXVIII*.

Page 131, 19th line, for " patomimic " read *pantomimic*.

Page 132, 12th line, for " patomimic " read *pantomimic*.

Page 205, 22d line, for " setting " read *sitting*.

Page 207, 8th line, for " loosing " read *loosening*.

PUBLISHER'S ANNOUNCEMENT.

In his "Letters upon the Æsthetic Education of Man," Schiller says: "I do not overlook the advantages to which the present race, regarded as a unity and in the balance of the understanding, may lay claim over what is best in the ancient world ; but it is obliged to engage in the contest as a compact mass, and measure itself as a whole against a whole. Who among the moderns could step forth, man against man, and strive with an Athenian for the prize of higher humanity? Whence comes this disadvantageous relation of individuals coupled with great advantages of the race? Why could the individual Greek be qualified as the type of his time, and why can no modern dare to offer himself as such? Because all-uniting nature imparted its forms to the Greek, and an all-dividing understanding gives our forms to us."

And, after he has traced back this contrast between the harmoniously educated man of antiquity and the one-sided culture of the man of the present to the difference between the mode of education of former times and that now prevalent, he demands for the individual, despite the general purpose he has to serve by a one-sided activity, the right for his own sake of a harmonious culture in all directions, thereby to bring the totality of his powers into exercise. He says this in the following words :

"But whatever may be the final profit for the totality of the world, of this distinct and special perfecting of the human faculties, it cannot be denied that this final aim of the universe, which devotes them to this kind of culture, is a cause of suffering, and a kind of malediction for individuals. I admit that the exercises of the gymnasium form athletic bodies ; but beauty is only developed by the free and equal play of the limbs. In the same way the tension of the isolated spiritual forces may make extraordinary men, but it is only the well-tempered equilibrium of these forces that can produce happy and accomplished men. * * But can it be true that man has to neglect himself for any end whatever ? Can nature snatch from us, for any end whatever, the perfection which is prescribed to us by the aim of reason ? It must be false that the perfecting of particular faculties renders the sacrifice of their totality necessary ; and even if the law of nature had imperiously this tendency, we must have the power to reform by a superior art this totality of our being, which art has destroyed."

Indeed, the exercise of this "superior art" is considered the great task of pedagogics since it has found a scientific basis. To educate man in the "totality of his nature," is the end which the greatest pedagogues have set themselves and their successors. Far enough as our age may still be from practically carrying out this idea, it is acknowledged in theory and set up as the ideal, never again, it is hoped, to be lost to mankind. Already the Germans possess a large literature pervaded by this idea ; the work having been, in this as in all other departments, divided and subdivided. For everywhere specialists work for the general end. In order, however, that such requisite, one-sided activity shall not prove misleading, each department must remain in conscious connection with the totality of the task. Let us here briefly mention the two principal points to be exemplified :

Education of the mind must never presume to thrive at the expense of that of the body ; and physical education must not forget that it can accomplish the highest ends only by aid of the mind. We have to treat to-day of a book which belongs in the latter category, a book on "Æsthetic Physical Culture," that physical culture which, to use Schiller's words, not only "develops athletic bodies but forms beauty by the free and equal play of the limbs."

Oskar Guttmann's book, "Æsthetic Physical Culture," a most valuable work which has for years been acknowledged to fill a great gap in this department of literature, has just been published in a second revised edition. On its first appearance, Dr. Feodor Wehl wrote: "A beautiful harmony is here struck between idealism and realism, which, understandingly called into life, can not remain without triumphant results." Spielhagen declared that he had "read the book repeatedly and with great interest, feeling true joy at the idea of the good it might do." In concluding its review, a Hamburg professional journal said: "In truth, our German literature possesses no work of this kind. That which lends it peculiar value is the scientific basis on which the author rests."

The necessity of asking the author, who resides in New York, to revise his book for republication in Germany, bears witness that his teachings have been verified by practice. His instructions are intended for two classes of people,— the cultured man in general and the actor in particular. His book, as he says in the preface to the second edition, "gives, in a strictly rational, scientific, and systematic manner, the means to æsthetically educate the body and its movements, and prepares the pupil to enter upon the study of mimic art." His system rests on the principle that gymnastics are the fundamental element of histrionic art; not, however, in the ordinary pedagogical (physical) sense, but with particular attention to plastic art and æsthetics. But inasmuch as mimic art is impossible without æsthetic gymnastics, so the latter are impossible without previous physical gymnastics. Who, in this connection, will not think of Goethe's words which, in his "Introduction to the Propylæum," he addresses to the artist: .

"The human form can not be comprehended merely by the contemplation of its surface. The interior must be laid bare, the parts separated, their union considered, their differences known, action and counter-action studied, the concealed, the ground, the foundation of the visible must be learned, if we would truly observe and imitate that which we see moving before our eyes in living waves, as one beautiful, undivided whole."

Like the sculptor who is to imitate truly the human form, so must man, who desires to use his frame correctly, "lay bare its interior to his consciousness, separate the parts, etc." In short, he must gain an insight into the anatomy of his body. Accordingly, Prof. Guttmann begins his work with "Anatomical and Physiological Principles," which he divides into three chapters,—"The Human Skeleton," "The Muscles," and "The Mechanism of the Limbs." "Physical Gymnastics" form the second part. The third, which is to be regarded as the principal portion of the book, treats of "Æsthetic Gymnastics," "The Plastic Art," and "The Mimic Art." Four other parts are added under the titles: "The Art of Dancing," "The Art of Fencing," "Main Principles of Dress," and "Application of the Rules to Common Life, the Salon and the Stage."

It may thus be seen how systematically the book is arranged, and how comprehensive it is. We are inclined to dwell with special emphasis on the practical use of that part which treats of the "Application of the Rules." In this country, more than in any other, does the need exist for such directions in *Æsthetic Physical Culture.* We have here no professional military class in whose officers our young men might find models of at least physical culture. Nor have we among us an aristocratic court circle whose members our ladies might deem just standards of demeanor. In our country the number daily grows of those, who, starting from humble surroundings, have become rapidly enriched, and, feeling urgent cause and the best will to demean themselves as cultured persons, yet are at a loss after what models to mould themselves. In democratic America, where every one possesses the right to call forth by self-instruction the best that is in him, and to constitute himself the "model," a work like that of Guttmann's ought to find a specially favorable reception.

Eighty-Seven Original Illustrations; Handsomely printed and bound; Price $2. postpaid. Address the Publisher,   EDGAR S. WERNER, Albany, N. Y.

FROM LEO KOFLER, TEACHER OF THE ART OF SINGING, NEW YORK.
[In his "The Old Italian School of Singing."]

We have arrived now at the last expedient of a singer's good style in singing ; namely, *the external demeanor of the body and the facial expression.* This subject ought to engage a singer's very careful attention and study. This was, hitherto, no easy matter. There was, to my knowledge, no work in existence that treated this subject fully and systematically from the singer's standpoint. It is true that in a number of books pertaining to the vocal and dramatic art, this subject has been ventilated ; but nowhere has it received the attention it deserves, except at the hands of Oskar Guttmann, in his excellent work, "Æsthetic Physical Culture." He treats this subject in his own practical and philosophical way, and I warmly commend his book to the faithful perusal of every student of vocal and dramatic art.

REVIEWS OF THE FIRST GERMAN EDITION.

[Friedrich Spielhagen in *Sonntagsblatt.*]

I have read the book over and over again, with great interest as I thought of the good it might do. Out of what rich source has the author drawn ! How clear is his proof that a stiff, awkward body cannot assume the various forms demanded for the portrayal of different characters ! It is certainly to be wished that this book will have a general circulation, for it will be found useful, not only to the actor and orator, but also to non-professional persons, who will learn in it what pertains to the drama and to oratory, and will be satisfied with nothing less than genuine art. But to those who choose the stage or the rostrum for a profession, the information contained in this book is indispensable. In it they better appreciate the meaning and importance of dramatic and oratorical art, and be shown what obstacles are to be overcome. They will learn that their profession is a noble one, and that to meet its requirements necessitates the earnest and persevering use of all their faculties. Those who believe they can accomplish everything through talent alone, without study, may exclaim, after examining the book, " The obstacles are insurmountable !" and make no further attempt. Such persons would do well to abandon the dramatic and oratorical profession, for energy and perseverance are qualities indispensable to the artist. Such persons as were born in unfavorable circumstances and could not receive proper culture, will find in this book the instruction they need,—what they must learn and how to learn it. They will be convinced that an actor or actress must have something more than mere physical beauty if he or she would be successful. Disciples of art, be diligent ! Show that you possess artistic tastes, and that you are sincerely striving to fulfill the mission to which you feel yourselves called !

[Leipzig *Journal.*]

This is the first exhaustive scientific treatise on æsthetic physical culture, and is designed not only for dramatic art but for all refined circles. This fact more than justifies our recommending the book—it makes it our *bounden duty* to do so.

[Hamburg *Theaterzeitung.*]

In fact, our German literature possesses no work of this kind. Its special value is the strictly scientific basis on which the author rests. The book is to be considered in a twofold manner,—from the general standpoint of a person of culture, and from the articular standpoint of a professional artist. The author proceeds from the right principle, namely, that every actor must first be a man of culture. In this respect, the scope of the book is a masterpiece. Prof. Guttmann's keen powers of observation, to which we had occasion to refer in reviewing his " Gymnastics of the Voice," are more strikingly manifested in "Æsthetic Physical Culture," and we urgently advise young persons of both sexes, who are anxious to improve themselves, to closely follow the teachings of both these books.

[Dresden *Gazette.*]

A first attempt, but so successful that it has fully accomplished its purpose. Indeed, in its clearness and thoroughness it surpasses all its predecessors.

[Hamburg *Reform.*]
In all the research and wisdom, in all the thoroughness and system continually shown in this work, the author steers clear of all pedantry, and nothing is farther from him than the idea that training alone will make an artist out of every grown person. The actor, like the poet, *must be born*—that is his unchangeable belief. But when mental endowment and dramatic fire exist, the body is the medium through which these must act, and to make it responsive in all its limbs, muscles and nerves, such study and such exercises as given in this book are indispensable. Part Third is the kernel of the whole book, and should be studied by all dramatic and oratorical students; not, however, before the first two parts have been thoroughly mastered. Indeed, it is a carefully graded text-book, no part of which can be omitted, if good results are desired. The book is designed for all cultured circles. Its study is greatly facilitated by the large number of wood cuts.

[Berlin *Music and Drama.*]
When it is remembered how often even prominent artists make themselves ridiculous by violations of the simplest laws of walking, speaking, and especially gesticulation, the details and exactness with which the author treats of these matters will be duly appreciated. From the discussion of the Hogarthian line of beauty, as the only sure basis for pleasing gestures, down to the directions for pantomimic reading and writing, there are rules and principles which every actor, singer and orator should carefully study. Every page contains something of value.

[Dresden *Constitutionelle Zeitung.*]
Guttmann's book does not tend to transgressions (of too frequent occurrence on the stage of the laws of noble proportions and beauty, nor does it lead to *mechanical* acting. On the contrary, it aims to correct these defects by recommending and giving the means to follow the maxim, more and more passing into forgetfulness, that "nature is to be copied in its beauty." We recommend Guttmann's book to the thorough study of all who wish to portray human sentiments.

[Dr. Feodor Wehl.]
Just now, when the tendency of the times is to view everything, even matters of art, with frivolous superficiality, special thanks are due the author, who so ably and successfully seeks to place dramatic art upon a scientific basis, and more in accord with the spirit and progress of the present day. A beautiful harmony is here struck between idealism and realism, which, understandingly called into life, cannot remain without triumphant results. May the entire dramatic profession, and all other persons of artistic vocations or natures, cordially welcome this book! By so doing they will themselves be benefited, and also promote dramatic and oratorical art.

[*Weserzeitung*, Bremen.]
Hitherto there has been no such a book, and for a pioneer one, "Æsthetic Physical Culture" comes surprisingly near the mark. From a thoroughly scientific basis, it develops, in clear, comprehensive language, and with numerous illustrations, the main rules for æsthetic attitudes and movements, as required in cultured society and in genuine dramatic art. The work is doubly valuable because it lays down as a fundamental principle that the training of an artist must be preceded by the training of a cultured person.

[Carlsruhe *Zeitung.*]
Two things are particularly required of a scientific work like "Æsthetic Physical Culture," viz., *thoroughness* and *utility*. These are found in Guttmann's book, and in the best manner. Another requisite is *intelligibility*, and this, too, is there. The author has diligently studied and mastered his subject, and has put his heart into the work, his own experience as an actor being of great service to him. The systematic arrangement of the book facilitates its study and makes it a guide to all. We wish for it an extended circulation, in order that people may attain unto greater æsthetic culture in all directions.

[Cologne *Zeitung.*]
"Æsthetic Physical Culture" is of great value to actors and orators, to theatrical managers and dramatic critics. It is also a guide and counsellor for refined society generally, especially for the rising generation, in questions of politeness and proper behavior.

www.ingramcontent.com/pod-product-compliance
Lightning Source LLC
Chambersburg PA
CBHW031749230426
43669CB00007B/555